Devolution
and Aging Policy

Devolution and Aging Policy has been co-published simultaneously as *Journal of Aging & Social Policy*, Volume 14, Numbers 3/4 2002.

The *Journal of Aging & Social Policy* Monographic "Separates"

Below is a list of " separates," which in serials librarianship means a special issue simultaneously published as a special journal issue or double-issue *and* as a "separate" hardbound monograph. (This is a format which we also call a "DocuSerial.")

"Separates" are published because specialized libraries or professionals may wish to purchase a specific thematic issue by itself in a format which can be separately cataloged and shelved, as opposed to purchasing the journal on an on-going basis. Faculty members may also more easily consider a "separate" for classroom adoption.

"Separates" are carefully classified separately with the major book jobbers so that the journal tie-in can be noted on new book order slips to avoid duplicate purchasing.

You may wish to visit Haworth's Website at . . .

http://www.HaworthPress.com

. . . to search our online catalog for complete tables of contents of these separates and related publications.

You may also call 1-800-HAWORTH (outside US/Canada: 607-722-5857), or Fax 1-800-895-0582 (outside US/Canada: 607-771-0012), or e-mail at:

getinfo@haworthpressinc.com

Devolution and Aging Policy, edited by Francis G. Caro, PhD, and Robert Morris, DSW (Vol. 14, No. 3/4, 2002). *Examines devolution–the decentralizing of service provision–and roles that state/local government and private organizations now play in addressing the needs of elders.*

Long-Term Care in the 21st Century: Perspectives from Around the Asia-Pacific Rim, edited by Iris Chi, DSW, Kalyani K. Mehta, PhD, and Anna L. Howe, PhD (Vol. 13, No. 2/3, 2001). *Discusses policies and programs for long-term care in the United States, Canada, Japan, Australia, Singapore, Hong Kong, and Taiwan.*

Advancing Aging Policy as the 21st Century Begins, edited by Francis G. Caro, PhD, Robert Morris, DSW, and Jill Norton (Vol. 11, No. 2/3, 2000). *"AN IDEAL TEXTBOOK for any graduate-level course on the aging population. Stands out among existing books on social problems and policies of the aging society. SUCCINCT AND TO THE POINT. A must-read for students, researchers, policy advocates, and policymakers." (Namkee G. Choi, PhD, Professor, Portland State University, Oregon)*

Public Policy and the Old Age Revolution in Japan, edited by Scott A. Bass, PhD, Robert Morris, DSW, and Masato Oka, MSc (Vol. 8, No. 2/3, 1996). *"Anyone seriously interested in the 21st Century and exploring means of adaptation to the revolution in longevity should read this book." (Robert N. Butler, MD, Director, International Longevity Center, The Mount Sinai Medical Center, New York)*

From Nursing Homes to Home Care, edited by Marie E. Cowart, DrPH, and Jill Quadagno, PhD (Vol. 7, No. 3/4, 1996). *"A compendium of research and policy information related to long-term care services, aging, and disability. Contributors address topics encompassing the risk of disability, access to and need for long-term care, and planning for a future long-term care policy." (Family Caregiver Alliance)*

International Perspectives on State and Family Support for the Elderly, edited by Scott A. Bass, PhD, and Robert Morris, DSW (Vol. 5, No. 1/2, 1993). *"The cross-cultural perspectives of the volume and the questions asked about what services are really needed and by whom they should be provided will be useful to the authors' intended audience in gerontological policymaking." (Academic Library Book Review)*

Devolution
and Aging Policy

Francis G. Caro, PhD
Robert Morris, DSW
Editors

Devolution and Aging Policy has been co-published simultaneously
as *Journal of Aging & Social Policy*, Volume 14, Numbers 3/4 2002.

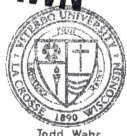

The Haworth Press, Inc.
New York • London • Oxford

Devolution and Aging Policy has been co-published simultaneously as *Journal of Aging & Social Policy*™, Volume 14, Numbers 3/4 2002.

The development, preparation, and publication of this work has been undertaken with great care. However, the publisher, employees, editors, and agents of The Haworth Press and all imprints of The Haworth Press, Inc., including The Haworth Medical Press® and Pharmaceutical Products Press®, are not responsible for any errors contained herein or for consequences that may ensue from use of materials or information contained in this work. Opinions expressed by the author(s) are not necessarily those of The Haworth Press, Inc. With regard to case studies, identities and circumstances of individuals discussed herein have been changed to protect confidentiality. Any resemblance to actual persons, living or dead, is entirely coincidental.

The Haworth Press, Inc., 10 Alice Street, Binghamton, NY 13904-1580 USA

Cover design by Jennifer M. Gaska

Library of Congress Cataloging-in-Publication Data

Devolution and aging policy / Francis G. Caro, Robert Morris, editors.
    p. cm.
    "Devolution and aging policy has been co-published simultaneously as Journal of aging & social policy, volume 14, numbers 3/4 2002."
    Includes bibliographical references and index.
    ISBN 0-7890-2080-7 (hardcover : alk. paper) – ISBN 0-7890-2081-5 (softcover : alk. paper)
    1. Aged–Government policy–United States. 2. Aged–Services for–United States. 3. Decentralization in government–United States. 4. Privatization–United States. I. Caro, Francis G., 1936- II. Morris, Robert, 1910- III. Journal of aging & social policy.
HV1461.D455 2002
362.6'0973–dc21
                                  2002156224

Indexing, Abstracting & Website/Internet Coverage

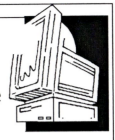

This section provides you with a list of major indexing & abstracting services. That is to say, each service began covering this periodical during the year noted in the right column. Most Websites which are listed below have indicated that they will either post, disseminate, compile, archive, cite or alert their own Website users with research-based content from this work. (This list is as current as the copyright date of this publication.)

Abstracting, Website/Indexing Coverage . . . . Year When Coverage Began

- *Abstracts in Anthropology* **1991**
- *Abstracts in Social Gerontology: Current Literature on Aging* **1991**
- *Academic Abstracts/CD-ROM* **1994**
- *Academic Search Elite (EBSCO)* **1995**
- *AgeInfo CD-ROM* **1995**
- *AgeLine Database* **1989**
- *Biology Digest (in print & online)* **1990**
- *Cambridge Scientific Abstracts <www.csa.com>* **1992**
- *caredata CD: The social and community care database*
  <www.scie.org.uk> **1996**
- *CINAHL (Cumulative Index to Nursing & Allied*
  Health Literature) <www.cinahl.com> **1996**
- *CNPIEC Reference Guide: Chinese National Directory*
  of Foreign Periodicals **1995**

(continued)

(continued)

*Special Bibliographic Notes related to special journal issues
(separates) and indexing/abstracting:*

- indexing/abstracting services in this list will also cover material in any "separate" that is co-published simultaneously with Haworth's special thematic journal issue or DocuSerial. Indexing/abstracting usually covers material at the article/chapter level.
- monographic co-editions are intended for either non-subscribers or libraries which intend to purchase a second copy for their circulating collections.
- monographic co-editions are reported to all jobbers/wholesalers/approval plans. The source journal is listed as the "series" to assist the prevention of duplicate purchasing in the same manner utilized for books-in-series.
- to facilitate user/access services all indexing/abstracting services are encouraged to utilize the co-indexing entry note indicated at the bottom of the first page of each article/chapter/contribution.
- this is intended to assist a library user of any reference tool (whether print, electronic, online, or CD-ROM) to locate the monographic version if the library has purchased this version but not a subscription to the source journal.
- individual articles/chapters in any Haworth publication are also available through the Haworth Document Delivery Service (HDDS).

Devolution
and Aging Policy

CONTENTS

PRIVATE SECTOR INITIATIVES

ABOUT THE EDITORS

Francis G. Caro, PhD, is Director of the Gerontology Institute and Professor of Gerontology at the University of Massachusetts Boston. His major interests in gerontology are home- and community-based long-term care and productive aging. Along with D. Frankfather and M. J. Smith, he is a co-author of *Family Care for the Elderly.* With A. Blank, he co-authored *Quality Impact of Home Care for the Elderly,* and with R. Morris and J. Hansan, *Personal Assistance: The Future of Home Care.* He also edited *Readings in Evaluation Research,* co-edited *Achieving a Productive Aging Society* with S. A. Bass and Y. P. Chen, and co-edited *Advancing Aging Policy as the 21st Century Begins* with R. Morris and J. Hansan. He is a member of the Gerontological Society of America.

Robert Morris, DSW, is a Senior Fellow for the Gerontology Institute at the University of Massachusetts Boston. He is also Professor Emeritus of the Heller School of Social Welfare at Brandeis University. He has authored or edited numerous books. His most recent book is *Social Work at the Millennium: Critical Reflections on the Future of the Profession* (co-authored with J. G. Gopps). He co-authored *Welfare Reform, 1996-2000* with J. E. Hansan and *Personal Assistance: The Future of Home Care* with Hansan and Francis G. Caro. He co-edited *Advancing Aging Policy as the 21st Century Begins* with Francis G. Caro and J. Norton. He is a Past President of the Gerontological Society of America.

INTRODUCTION

Devolution and Aging Policy

Francis G. Caro, PhD

Gerontology Institute, University of Massachusetts

Robert Morris, DSW

Senior Fellow, Gerontology Institute, University of Massachusetts

DEVOLUTION: AN OVERVIEW

Around the world, the ground rules are being questioned about the role of national governments in addressing domestic needs. During the twentieth century in countries throughout the world, central governments assumed major responsibilities for a wide variety of human needs. Whether the concern was income security, health, housing, or education, interventions were premised upon convictions that a strong public sector role was essential and that major involvement of national governments was needed. The role of national governments in these initiatives varied greatly. In some instances, national governments carried full responsibility, from financing to service administration. In other in-

[Haworth co-indexing entry note]: "Devolution and Aging Policy." Caro, Francis G., and Robert Morris. Co-published simultaneously in *Journal of Aging & Social Policy* (The Haworth Press, Inc.) Vol. 14, No. 3/4, 2002, pp. 1-14; and: *Devolution and Aging Policy* (ed: Francis G. Caro, and Robert Morris) The Haworth Press, Inc., 2002, pp. 1-14. Single or multiple copies of this article are available for a fee from The Haworth Document Delivery Service [1-800-HAWORTH, 9:00 a.m. - 5:00 p.m. (EST). E-mail address: getinfo@haworthpressinc.com].

10.1300/J031v14n03_01

stances, the role of national governments is limited with other entities carrying major responsibilities. In some cases, the role of national governments was limited, for example, to financing and regulation, with regional governments, local governments, private organizations, and even private individuals carrying other responsibilities. In other cases, the role of national governments has been limited to nurturing innovation and dissemination of information. In these cases, national governments help to find solutions to problems but expect that other levels of government or private organizations will solve the problems.

More recently, a significant pattern has emerged in many countries of the shifting of responsibilities away from national governments to regional and local governments and the shifting of responsibilities from the public sector to the private sector. The term "devolution" refers to the pattern of decentralizing governmental responsibilities. Typically, the term refers to a transfer of responsibilities from national authorities to regional or local authorities.

Devolution and privatization are related themes. Privatization shifts responsibilities from the public to the private sector. Both devolution and privatization imply weaker responsibilities for national governments.

The arguments about the relative merits of public and private problem solving, centralization and decentralization of governmental responsibilities are deeply rooted in the political thought in this country and elsewhere. In a recent scholarly book on privatization, for example, George Liebmann traces the debate about decentralization to the writings of Alexis De Tocqueville (Liebmann, 2000). John Donahue makes the point eloquently:

> The shift in government's center of gravity away from Washington and toward the states . . . reflects an uncommon pause in an endless American argument over the balance between nation and state. That argument got underway when the Framers gathered in Philadelphia to launch a second attempt at nationhood, after less than a decade's dismal experience under the feeble Articles of Confederation. The Constitution they crafted was a compromise between those who wanted to strengthen the ties among essentially autonomous states, and those who sought to establish a new nation to supersede the states as the locus of the commonwealth.

In the United States in recent years, the single greatest focus for devolution has been the transformation of income security protections for poor families. The federal Aid to Families With Dependent Children

Program has been replaced by the Temporary Assistance to Needy Families program. The new program provides states with greater responsibility and greater discretion. The federal government has set limits on its financial participation; states have been granted greater freedom in administering programs.

In the United States, devolution has unfolded incrementally and partially. The dramatic changes in assistance to poor families are an exception. In other sectors, changes have come more slowly. The heightened concern with terrorism, in fact, has lead to a rediscovery of the importance of a strong role for the federal government–at least with respect to defense against terrorism.

In other countries, devolution involves very different issues. In Great Britain and Spain, for example, devolution involves the shifting of a wide variety of responsibilities to regional governments. In Great Britain, devolution has involved the establishment of new legislative bodies for Scotland and Wales.

In this collection of articles, the focus is on the locus of responsibility for initiatives to address the needs of older people at a time when national governments are consolidating responsibilities for the programs in which they are involved, shifting responsibilities to other units of government, and resisting new initiatives.

The locus of problem solving is a persistent focus for debate. The major themes in these debates are generic. Advocates for public interventions often base their cases on the need for universal access that can only be achieved through public involvement. They also argue that the unique taxing and/or regulatory authority of the public sector is needed to solve problems. Critics of public interventions often challenge the need for universal access and complain about taxes and regulations as unjustified infringements on individual freedom.

Interventions by national governments are attractive when issues are national in scope and when there is potential for national policies and programs to reach entire populations. The movement of people, ideas, and goods within countries often invites national interventions. When goods are distributed nationally, for example, national consumer protection measures are likely to be more effective than local measures. When policy differences among states are great enough to encourage internal migration to take advantage of services or tax policies, proposals for uniform national policies can be anticipated from states adversely affected by internal migration.

On the other hand, the development of national interventions is difficult when there are major regional differences in political philosophy.

Further, in their administration, national interventions often experience difficulties in responding to unique local conditions. In contrast, state and local governments are often seen to be capable of moving more quickly and sensitively than national governments in addressing local needs.

In the United States, the federal government plays a stronger role in health and welfare programs to meet needs of older people than it does in interventions to assist children. Both Social Security and Medicare are financed entirely by the federal government and are major items in the federal budget. Social Security is also entirely administered by the federal government. Medicare can be considered a public-private partnership since the federal government provides the financing, insurance companies process claims, and most of the care is provided by private organizations and individuals. Although the Supplemental Security Income program (SSI) provides opportunities for state supplementation, SSI is also a federally financed and administered program. The federal government also plays a major role in contributing to financing of the Medicaid program, which is important for nursing home financing and supplementary medical insurance for low-income elders. At the same time, some of the public interventions in the United States on behalf of older people rely much more heavily on state and local governments. The aging services network illustrates the point. The federal government through the Administration has established a framework that calls for State Units on Aging and Area Agencies on Aging within states. Federal legislation provides the aging service network with a very broad mandate but very little funding. The federal expectation is that federal funds will be generously supplemented by state and local funds (Gelfand, 1999).

In contrast, public education, the intervention with the greatest importance for young people, is largely funded through local property taxes. States often play a major role in supplementing local property taxes. Even though presidential politics sometimes focuses on elementary and secondary education, the role of the federal government in financing elementary and secondary education is minor.

In countries throughout the world, serious challenges have been posed to some of the national health and welfare interventions that were developed in the middle of the twentieth century. In some countries, proposals have been put forward for privatization of services that have been offered by public agencies. In other cases, proposals are being heard for shifting of responsibility for program policies, financing, and administration from national governments to state and local governments. In other cases, national governments are simply deflecting proposals for new interventions.

The reasons for the challenges to strong national programs are varied. Some of the reaction stems from resistance to taxes. Particularly in the case of entitlement programs that serve older people, the growth in the numbers of people who receive benefits has added greatly to the expense. In the case of health insurance programs, the costs are growing rapidly not only because of the increases in numbers served but also because of higher costs of increasingly sophisticated services.

Some of the challenges come from those who prefer private to public problem solving. In part, this theme reflects a preference for private markets in which those interested in a service seek it in a market that rewards creativity and competitiveness. The preference for market solutions may also reflect reduced sympathy for vulnerable individuals who cannot afford private solutions.

In the United States, the strong role that the federal government developed in a variety of domestic issues between 1935 and 1975 can also be viewed as a historical aberration. Through most of its history, the United States government has played a relatively minor role on health and welfare matters. Until the Great Depression, health and welfare were considered state responsibilities. The massive widespread and sustained suffering triggered by the Great Depression provided a rationale for an unprecedented involvement of the federal government in addressing domestic problems. World War II and the Cold War provided a rationale for continuing a strong federal role. It can be argued that, between the end of the Cold War and the terrorist attacks in September 2001, the country had returned to more normal times in which citizens looked less often to the public sector for problem solving and preferred their public interventions to be at state and local levels rather than a federal level.

Other reasons for the interest in reducing the role of the federal government in domestic programs can be offered. Some federal interventions were welcome in principle but proved to be so clumsy in their implementation that they invited a search for public interventions designed, financed, and administered closer to home.

Another potential reason is that the costs of the major federal programs are so great that the federal government has its hands full in sustaining its commitments to those programs. Just three programs of major importance to older people, Social Security, Medicare, and Medicaid accounted for over 40% of federal outlays in 1998 (Wildavsky & Caiden, 2001, pp. 188-189). All three programs pose major financial challenges for the federal government. Social Security is a looming problem because the taxes paid by workers and employers and the interest generated by the taxes are not sufficient to cover the benefits that have been promised. Similarly, the special payroll taxes to finance Medicare will not be sufficient in the long run to finance benefits. Medicaid is a major financial challenge because of expanding demand for services and pressures to make upward adjustments in reimbursement rates to assure the continued willingness of providers to participate. An argument can be made that the federal government should concentrate its efforts on a limited number of the major programs and leave other problems to be addressed elsewhere.

In the United States, many social welfare advocates remain convinced about the need for a strong federal government role in addressing human needs. They are skeptical about what can be accomplished through programs administered by state and local governments or the private sector. Many remain convinced that globalization of economic life, immigration, internal migration, national and international travel, the national and international nature of contemporary systems of communication and cultural life, the potential for international transmission of diseases, and the involvement of the United States in political disputes throughout the world all point to a need for an even stronger role of the federal government in domestic matters. Some also see the federal government as the guarantor of individual rights when minorities are disregarded or oppressed at a local level. Others see the federal government as the protector of vulnerable individuals in places where local resources are insufficient to provide adequate public services. Others look to the federal government as a source of protection in hard financial times because of its greater financial resources and greater borrowing power.

The realities of federal-state relationships may be more complex than is suggested by the ideological arguments about devolution and privatization. Michael Sparer (1999) argues that over the past 60 years the growth of both federal and state involvement in health care overshadows the arguments about the division of labor between the federal government and the states. In the health policy arena, he argues that the federal government is expanding its health policy agenda rather than delegating more authority to states. Sparer sees the intergovernmental partnership as becoming more complex rather than one in which the overall federal role is declining.

THE ARTICLES ON DEVOLUTION AND AGING POLICY

The articles in this collection concern efforts to address needs of elders in a context of diminished expectations of the federal government. Some of the papers are concerned with issues in which the federal government is less active than it was in the past. Other papers speak to new issues being addressed at a state or local level. We have organized the articles based on the sectors they address; we distinguish among federal-state collaborations, strictly state or local initiatives, and private efforts. We also distinguish among issues in implementation of established programs, innovation within established programs, and new initiatives. We begin with three papers that examine the implementation of established programs involving federal and state collaboration. The second group consisting of two papers is concerned with innovation within established programs. The third category, with a single paper, examines a federal demonstration designed to stimulate service development within states. A fourth group of papers considers public sector interventions that have arisen at the state or local level without the participation of the federal government. The fifth group consisting of three papers examines interventions that are entirely private.

Implementation of Established Federal-State Programs

Medicaid Financing of Long-Term Care. Medicaid, the major public means of financing long-term care services in the United States, is a collaboration between the federal government and the states. The federal government provides at least 50% of the financing and specifies that some core services are covered; states decide what services are to be covered (beyond those required by the federal government), establish the eligibility of providers for reimbursement, and set reimbursement rates. In his article, Edward Alan Miller documents the variability in the manner in which states use Medicaid to finance long-term care services for residents. Miller illustrates how some states effectively use Medicaid to make unusually strong long-term care options available to residents; however, he also provides evidence of how low-income people with functional disabilities are much less adequately served by other states–thus raising questions whether a stronger federal role is needed to assure minimally acceptable levels of service.

Upgrading Older Workers' Skills. Focusing on economic development issues in Massachusetts, Peter Doeringer, Andrew Sum, and David Terkla make a case for public sector intervention to upgrade the skills of older workers. By examining demographic patterns, the authors show that the state's economy will be increasingly reliant on older workers. Anticipated shortages of skilled workers point to a need for upgrading of skills for those already in the workforce. The federal Workforce Investment Act of 1998 provides enormous discretion to state and local employment and training agencies. The paper outlines the enormous challenges faced by state and local agencies in investing public resources wisely for the upgrading of workforce skills. They point to the importance of a political commitment to financing training at adequate levels and to systematic evaluation to assure that training resources are efficiently invested.

The Long-Term Care Ombudsman Program. In their article, Andrew Whitford and Jeff Yates show how devolution can lead to inequities in the administration of a federal program that serves vulnerable elders. The inequities they document result not simply from the different financial capacity or generosity of states in matching federal funds but from their ability to recruit volunteers. The Long-Term Care Ombudsman Program is a federal program designed to protect consumers of long-term care services from abuse and to advocate for quality of care. Like other programs authorized by the Older Americans Act, the federal financial contribution is modest. The scope of the program in each state depends greatly on the manner in which states choose to supplement the federal resources. Since state financial contributions also tend to be modest, the relative strength of state programs rests heavily upon the extent to which volunteers are used. Whitford and Yates show that the number of volunteers used in the states is associated with a social capital, a broad indicator of the extent of civic engagement. In other words, in states with greater civic engagement, the volunteer component of the Long-Term Care Ombudsman program tends to be larger. The greater the extent of civic engagement, the more effectively the program is able to serve long-term care recipients. Since social capital has been declining in the United States, programs like the Long-Term Care Ombudsman Program that depend heavily on volunteers face an uphill struggle in maintaining their effectiveness. The format of the Long-Term Care Ombudsman program invites holding state officials accountable for the relative strength of their programs. However, the forces that affect the civic engagement that underlies volunteering are both local and national. The research invites questions about the extent to which both federal and state policymakers are sensitive to the forces that underlie volunteering and are committed to assuring the program's effectiveness even when the availability of volunteers is sharply limited.

Innovation Within Established Federal-State Programs

The Partnership Long-Term Care Insurance Program. In their article, Mark Meiners, Hunter McKay, and Kevin Mahoney call upon two contemporary themes, devolution and privatization, in their account of the Partnership Demonstrations. The context for these demonstrations was the reluctance of the federal government to provide universal long-term care financing in a social insurance framework. Through the Medicaid program, the federal government and state governments share the cost of financing long-term care for the poor. While the system provides a welcome safety net, it creates an awkward situation for middle-income elders. By spending down (or otherwise depleting) their assets, middle-income elders can establish eligibility for Medicaid-financed nursing home care. In doing so, however, those elders largely lose control over their financial affairs and give up their ability to pass on assets to their heirs. The Partnership Program was established with support of the Robert Wood Johnson Foundation to encourage middle-income families to purchase private long-term care insurance. To the extent that individuals maintain Partnership policies, their assets are protected while Medicaid pays for their long-term care. Partnership Programs have been established in Connecticut, Indiana, New York, and California. At a minimum, the Partnerships represent a creative collaboration among the federal government, state governments, private insurers, and a major foundation that provides elders with an improved option for coping with the risks of long-term care expenses. While the Partnerships show that complex, constructive interventions are possible, the experience also illustrates the fragility of these arrangements. While Partnership policies have been gaining consumer acceptance, especially in California, a change in the federal authorizing legislation has discouraged replication of the Partnership Program in additional states.

Consumer-Directed Care Demonstrations. Lori Simon-Rusinowitz and colleagues are concerned with a shifting of responsibility within Medicaid-funded personal assistance programs. Here, the responsibility for directing care that previously was invested entirely in case managers has been transferred substantially to consumers. The community care demonstrations take place in New Jersey, Florida, and Arkansas. The clients who choose the self-direction model are authorized to hire and supervise their own personal assistance workers. Self-direction not only enables clients to obtain a greater quantity of personal assistance but enables them to hire neighbors and relatives as personal assistants. The demonstrations are useful in showing not only that a substantial proportion of clients are interested in self-direction; they are also successful in hiring and supervising their own personal assistants. Further, arrangements can be put in place to assure protection to the rights of these private contractors to being paid regularly, to have Social Security payments made on their behalves, and to obtain workman's compensation protection.

In short, the Consumer-Directed Care Demonstration provides greater leverage to consumers of services without making any basic change in the division of responsibility between the federal government and state governments in the administration of these programs.

A Federal Demonstration to Stimulate Service Development Within States

The National Alzheimer's Disease Service Demonstration. This demonstration is another example of a federal initiative that has been useful in stimulating service development in some underserved areas, but has left the underlying problems to be addressed by state or local government, the private sector, or families. In their article, Rhonda Montgomery, Tracy Karner, and Karl Kosloski provide an overview of a demonstration program designed to help states with program development, service delivery, and information dissemination to help families caring for elders with Alzheimer's disease. The demonstration was successful in stimulating development of support services that reached and were welcomed by the families. However, states varied in the strength of their service development efforts. They also varied in the stability and longevity of their programs. In some cases, the demonstrations led states to make financial commitments to sustain the services. Montgomery, Karner, and Kosloski found that the program reinforced inequalities among states; states and communities with the weakest infrastructure had less capacity to take advantage of the program. The authors also express concern that while the federal role in stimulating service development has been welcome, the initiative has been the means through which Congress has deflected the major responsibility for care of elders with Alzheimer's disease back to states, communities, and, ultimately, to families.

Public Sector, State, and Local Initiatives

Property Tax Work-Off Programs for Seniors. Kristin Kiesel provides a case study of a local initiative that combines volunteer public community service by elders with modest property tax credits. Typically, the Senior Tax Work-Off programs that have been introduced in the past decade in over 50 Massachusetts cities and towns provide $500 in property tax credits to seniors who work for their towns for 100 hours. Making this program particularly interesting is that it was introduced in Massachusetts and has spread *without* the assistance of federal or state government or a private foundation. The approach was introduced by the Council on Aging in Chelmsford, MA. Through its own resources, the council devised the program on the basis of what it learned about a more restricted program offered by a school district in Colorado. The program benefits from some supportive Massachusetts legislation, but the viability of the program does not depend on state support. Discussion of senior volunteer programs often begins and ends with federal initiatives. Kiesel's paper provides an account of a volunteer program that arose at the grassroots level and has spread rapidly to other jurisdictions.

A State Public Education Program on Long-Term Care Financing. Sanjay Pandey provides a case study of compensatory federalism, that is, an increased activity by state government to make up for a reduced federal role. He provides an account of an unsuccessful campaign mounted by the Maryland state government to encourage citizens to take responsibility for financing their own long-term care planning. (In another era, the federal government might have provided leadership for this campaign.) Pandey seeks to explain why the long-term care campaign failed to gain momentum. He attributes the lack of success to insufficient support from top leadership; an inability of the responsible state agency to motivate other organizations to participate; and an excessive reliance on external stakeholders whose support was uncertain. Pandey illustrates some of the skills in political analysis and organizing that are essential if state governments are to provide effective leadership in public education campaigns.

Naturally Occurring Retirement Community-Supportive Service Program. Patricia Pine and Vanderlyn Pine describe a supportive service demonstration program developed by New York state to address the needs of those aging in place in apartment buildings or housing complexes for low- or moderate-income people. The focus of the demonstration is on older residents of housing that was not originally built for older people but is now dominated by long-time residents who have aged in place. The demonstrations provide care management, personal assistance, and health services. In an earlier period, congregate housing for the elderly constructed with federal support might have served many of the elders served by this initiative. Thus, the paper illustrates a state program that addresses an elder service need that emerged during a period in which the federal government has drastically curtailed its involvement in expansion of the supply of service-assisted housing for low- and moderate-income elders.

Information Technology to Assist Elders. In her paper, Carolyn Shrewsbury shows the potential of recent developments in information technology to improve the lives of elders. In another era, we might have expected the federal government to be active in promoting access to information technology for disadvantaged elders and those who serve elders. We might have expected the federal government to be particularly interested in information technology for rural elders as a way of compensating for geographic isolation. Shrewsbury shows that in this era states have the potential to be important players in drawing on information technology to assist elders. Shrewsbury discusses the role of states in five aspects of information technology policy: obtaining access, minimizing inequities in access, developing information management systems, providing information over the Internet, and maintaining privacy. Shrewsbury finds evidence of constructive developments in each sector. Predictably, the strength of these developments varies from one state to another. She holds open the possibility of an integrated national policy when the issues are better understood.

Private Sector Initiatives

Consumer Cooperative Association for Elders. In the only international paper in this collection, Masato Oka describes a consumer cooperative that has developed in Kanagawa Prefecture in Japan to provide services for the elderly. The co-op arose out of a larger cooperative association that has attempted to develop a total life support system at a neighborhood level. The co-op organizes homemaker collectives that offer a variety of services to elders on a fee basis. The co-op provides not only homemaking services, but also home-delivered meals and transportation. The co-op has also opened a residential development that includes an adult day care center and has become important both as a source of employment opportunities and for the services that it provides to elders. The co-op's ability to attract and retain customers is a reflection both of the decline in the capacity of families in Japan to provide long-term care and dissatisfaction with service programs offered by the government. To date, the co-op has proved viable both with respect to attracting workers and customers. From a devolution perspective, the Japanese co-op is significant as a private nonprofit initiative that emerged without government support in response to dissatisfaction with public sector approaches.

The Kaiser Permanente Manifesto 2005. Walter Leutz, Merwyn Greenlick, Lucy Nonnenkamp, and Richard della Penna discuss an ambitious private service coordination effort covering 32 sites. The Kaiser Permanente Manifesto 2005 demonstration sought to integrate traditional health care provided by HMOs with existing home- and community-based long-term care services. In the recent past, the federal government might have provided incentives to state governments to mount the kind of broad project attempted by Kaiser Permanente. The paper shows that a good deal was accomplished through the demonstration. At the same time, the demonstration was less successful in reaching the "unprofitable" populations that have been primary targets for publicly-financed interventions.

Privately Financed Community Care: Age Concerns. Focusing on long-term community care for elders who are above the income eligibility limits for publicly-financed community care programs, David Stoesz provides an account of a private effort to address a need that has received little recognition. Most of the attention to community care in the United States has been given to programs that serve poor elders on the basis of public subsidies. Some would prefer that the community care programs developed for low-income elders be extended to all elders. In light of the cost of community care, the growing numbers of more affluent elders who can pay for care themselves, and the absence of a strong political constituency asking for a social insurance program to cover long-term care, it is not likely that middle- and upper-income elders will have access to the publicly-funded community care programs.

Stoesz describes Age Concerns, a private agency in San Diego that has grown incrementally to provide privately-financed community care. Age Concerns is of interest because it is relatively unusual. Age Concerns offers care management and a menu of services that includes homemaking, personal care, transportation, and shopping. Clients live in a variety of settings including private homes, assisted living, and even nursing homes. Clients are served on a sustained basis–typically four years. Age Concerns delivers substantial services; clients are paying an average of $5,000 per month, an amount that is in the range of what nursing home care costs. Clearly, Age Concerns has found a way to compete effectively with both assisted living facilities and freelance personal assistance workers. The paper demonstrates that in this instance a viable community-care program has emerged that provides substantial personal assistance over an extended period to the self-pay market.

CONCLUSION

The tendency of central governments to concentrate on a limited set of needs of the elderly, shift some responsibilities to states, and deflect new problems to other entities has created enormous opportunities for problem solving by state governments, local governments, and private organizations. This collection of articles suggests some of the possibilities. Devolution creates abundant opportunities for creativity in addressing local needs.

Broadly speaking, the devolution movement can be considered a large informal experiment. To the extent that the experiment is judged to be successful, devolution will flourish. To the extent that the experiment fails, national programs may come back into favor. Devolution also invites systematic investment in evaluation. The creative interventions that show great promise when they are introduced may not stand up well in the long run if they are subject to thorough evaluation. The evaluation is too important to be left to chance. In the current environment, national foundations without an ideological stake in the devolution movement are in the best position to sponsor wide-ranging assessments of devolution as it affects elder concerns.

REFERENCES

Donahue, J. D. (1997). "The devil in devolution." *American Prospect.* http://www.prospect.org/print/V8/32/donahue-j.html.

Gelfand, D. E. (1999). *The Aging Network: Programs and Services.* Fifth Edition. New York: Springer.

Liebmann, G. W. (2000). *Solving Problems Without Large Government: Devolution, Fairness, and Equality.* Westport, CT: Praeger.

Sparer, M. S. (1999). Myths and misunderstandings: Health policy, the devolution revolution, and the push for privatization. *American Behavioral Scientist, 43*(1), 138-154.

Wildavsky, A. & Caiden, N. (2001). *The New Politics of the Budgetary Process.* Fourth Edition. New York: Addison, Wesley, Longman.

IMPLEMENTATION OF ESTABLISHED FEDERAL-STATE PROGRAMS

State Discretion and Medicaid Program Variation in Long-Term Care: When Is Enough, Enough?

Edward Alan Miller, MPA, MA

University of Michigan

SUMMARY. Although federal statutes and regulations establish the broad parameters within which state Medicaid programs operate, the federal government grants states substantial discretion over Medicaid and Medicaid-funded long-term care. An appreciation of resulting cross-state variation in Medicaid program characteristics, however, has been lacking in the ongoing debate over whether the federal government should further devolve responsibility for caring for the poor and disabled elderly to the states. To better inform this discussion, therefore, this article documents considerable variation, not only in terms of Medicaid program spending and recipients, but also in terms of strategies chosen to reform long-term care services and financing. Since there is little doubt that states take full advantage of current levels of discretion, advocates of devolution may want to reassess their views to consider whether existing

[Haworth co-indexing entry note]: "State Discretion and Medicaid Program Variation in Long-Term Care: When Is Enough, Enough?" Miller, Edward Alan. Co-published simultaneously in *Journal of Aging & Social Policy* (The Haworth Press, Inc.) Vol. 14, No. 3/4, 2002, pp. 15-35; and: *Devolution and Aging Policy* (ed: Francis G. Caro, and Robert Morris) The Haworth Press, Inc., 2002, pp. 15-35. Single or multiple copies of this article are available for a fee from The Haworth Document Delivery Service [1-800-HAWORTH, 9:00 a.m. - 5:00 p.m. (EST). E-mail address: getinfo@haworthpressinc.com].

10.1300/J031v14n03_02

variation has resulted in inequities addressable only through more, not less, federal involvement. *[Article copies available for a fee from The Haworth Document Delivery Service: 1-800-HAWORTH. E-mail address: <getinfo@haworthpressinc.com> Website: <http://www.HaworthPress.com> © 2002 by The Haworth Press, Inc. All rights reserved.]*

KEYWORDS. Medicaid, long-term care, elderly, devolution, federalism

INTRODUCTION

Federal statutes and regulations establish the broad parameters within which state Medicaid programs operate, while federal administrative review and the courts ultimately determine whether or not particular state actions fall within the purview of federal guidelines. That the federal government might want to exercise vigilance in its oversight of the Medicaid program should come as no surprise, given its substantial role in financing the program. In 2000, for example, the federal government paid for 56.7% of total program expenditures of $194.7 billion, including $38.0 billion for long-term care services (CMS, 2002a). As a grant-in-aid, moreover, Medicaid has grown exponentially over the years. From just 14% of federal grant-in-aid monies in 1975, it has become the largest program, accounting for nearly 40% of the $271.3 billion in federal grant-in-aid monies flowing to the states in 1999. Neither transportation (10%), education (4%), Temporary Assistance for Needy Families (6%), nor food stamp/child nutrition programs (5%) represent a larger share (Kaiser Commission, 1999).

States are also subject to a large volume of federal regulation. The Medicaid section of the U.S. Code is now more than 500 pages, compared to 10 pages for the original statute. In addition, states are subject to more than 300 pages in the *Code of Federal Regulations*, not to mention other directives and guidelines promulgated by the Centers for Medicare and Medicaid Services (CMS), which oversees the program (Thompson, 1998). To facilitate CMS oversight, moreover, Medicaid rules require that a single agency assume responsibility for administering the program in each state. This agency, which is usually a state welfare, health, or human resources agency, may in turn contract with other entities to perform program functions.

Although the federal government retains a right to intervene as circumstances dictate, it grants states substantial control over Medicaid and Medicaid-funded long-term care, not only in terms of spending and recipients served, but also in terms of available strategies to reform the delivery and financing of long-term care services. In addition to expanding managed care and home- and community-based services options, for example, states may rely on a succession of more traditional strategies related to benefits, providers, eligibility, and reimbursement. An appreciation of existing variation, however, has been lacking in the ongoing debate over whether the federal government should further devolve responsibility for caring for the poor and disabled elderly to the states. To better inform this discussion, therefore, we first review national- and state-level trends in Medicaid spending and recipients. This is followed by a more extended examination of state long-term care reform options and the substantial discretion states posses in choosing the particular strategies that they do. We continue by discussing the history of Medicaid program changes and by reviewing arguments in favor of and against devolution. We conclude by laying out the implications of state Medicaid program variation for this debate.

MEDICAID AND THE ELDERLY BY THE NUMBERS: A NATION'S EYE VIEW

National Long-Term Care Spending

In 1998, overall spending on long-term care in the United States amounted to $117 billion or 11.5% of all personal health care spending (HCFA, 2000). Most long-term care is funded by the Medicaid program (39.0%) and by individuals and their families (29.5%), with Medicare (17.8%) and private health insurance (7.4%) playing much smaller roles. The majority of long-term care expenditures (75% or $87.8 billion) were spent on nursing homes and intermediate care facilities for the mentally retarded (ICF-MR). At 46.2% and 32.5%, respectively, Medicaid and out-of-pocket payments paid for the provision of most of these services. Home health care, on the other hand, constitutes 25% or $29.3 billion of total long-term care spending. At 17.1%, Medicaid's role in funding home health care is smaller than that of Medicare (35.6%) and out-of-pocket contributions (20.5%).

Medicaid and the Elderly

Close to 4 million of Medicaid's 40.6 million recipients in 1998 were ages 65 or older (CMS, 2002b). Though only 9.75% of beneficiaries, the elderly consumed close to 28.5% of program expenditures in 1998. At $10,243, per enrollee payments for the elderly well exceeded that of most other eligibility groups, including the blind and disabled ($9,097), children ($1,117), non-disabled adults ($1,876), and foster care children ($3,584). Overall, the program spent $40.6 billion on aged recipients, of which approximately 64.6% ($26.2 billion) and 10.1% ($4.1 billion) went toward nursing facility and home care, respectively. At $3.8 billion or 9.4% of total spending, prescription drugs, which are often needed for the management of chronic illnesses and conditions, was the third largest category of spending for the aged. In contrast, the three largest categories of services for children and non-disabled adult recipients were inpatient hospitals, physicians, and prepaid health services.

One reason Medicaid spends so much more on long-term care for the elderly is that they are more likely to suffer from the chronic ailments and disabilities that requires long-term care. Defined as a need for assistance with activities of daily living, one report estimates that more than half of the 12.1 million Americans with long-term care needs were age 65 or over in 1995 (Niefield, O'Brien, & Feder, 1999) even though elderly people constituted less than 13% of the population that year. While the elderly accounted for 48.1% of community residents with long-term care needs (5.1 million), they accounted for 87% of nursing home residents (1.3 million).

Current Trends in Medicaid Spending

Medicaid long-term care spending reached $67.7 billion or 34.8% of total Medicaid expenditures of $194.3 billion in 2000. While 26.8% of Medicaid long-term care spending was devoted to community-based services (i.e., personal care, home- and community-based waiver services, and home health), 73.2% was directed toward institutional services (i.e., nursing home care plus ICF-MR) (Burwell, 2001). Between 1988 and 2000 total Medicaid and Medicaid long-term care grew at annual compound rates of 11.7% and 9.4%, respectively. Though high, these figures mask a particularly dramatic compound annual rate of growth of 27.8% for home- and community-based waiver expenditures during this time period. They also mask an especially explosive period between 1988 and 1992 when Medicaid grew at an average annual rate of 22.1%, and Medicaid long-term care grew at 14.0%. Spending has since slowed, however. Between 1993 and 1999, average annual increases in total Medicaid and Medicaid long-term care expenditures dropped to 6.9% and 7.2%, respectively.

Analysts attribute the trend toward greater Medicaid expenditures earlier in the decade to the convergence of a variety of factors, including medical price inflation, extraordinary growth in Disproportionate Share Hospital (DSH) payments to facilities serving disproportionate shares of indigent beneficiaries, and increases in the number of recipients, including low-income adults and children as well as the elderly and disabled (Bruen & Holahan, 1999). Increases in health care utilization for people with higher needs (e.g., pregnant women, AIDS patients) and economic recession also played a role. Since then, the rate of growth has slowed for a number of reasons, including federal legislation, which curtailed state use of DSH payments, a slow down in enrollment growth, especially among pregnant women and children, and lowering of growth in spending per enrollee, possibly resulting from lower medical price inflation, rapid increases in managed care enrollment, and other economic changes. Lower enrollment of low-income adults and children combined with steady enrollment of aged beneficiaries and growing enrollment of blind and disabled individuals in recent years have led spending on long-term care and prescription drugs to grow more quickly than other services.

Future Trends in Medicaid Spending

Between 2000 and 2020, the number of individuals 65 and older is projected to increase by approximately 50% (from 35.5 to 52.6 million), while the number of individuals 85 and older is projected to increase by 26% (from 4.6 to 5.8 million, reaching more than 14 million by 2050) (The Lewin Group, 2000). At the same time, the number of disabled elderly persons with at least one ADL or IADL limitation is expected to grow by 42% (from 5.2 to 7.4 million), in large part due to the dramatic growth in the number of individuals 85 and older. Well aware that demographic expenditures indicate significant growth among the oldest old and that growing ranks of the population will be chronically ill and disabled, the Congressional Budget Office (CBO) has projected expenditures on long-term care services nearly to double from $123.1 billion in 2000 to $207.3 billion in 2020 (CBO, 1999). Long-term expenditures by the Medicaid program, in particular, are expected to grow from $43.3 to $75.4 billion during this time period. CBO expects Medicaid to account for one-third of the growth in federal spending between 1997 and 2030 (CBO, 1997).

MEDICAID AND THE ELDERLY BY THE NUMBERS:
A STATE'S EYE VIEW

Variation in Recipients and Spending

The federal government grants states significant flexibility in design-ing and administering the Medicaid program, resulting in tremendous variation in program spending among the states (Holahan & Liska, 1998). The following 1998 statistics, the last year for which detailed data are available, are illustrative of this variation (CMS, 2002b).

- The percentage of elderly recipients ranged from 4.4% in both Washington and Utah to 14.6% in Pennsylvania and 16.7% in North Dakota.
- The proportion of total payments for the elderly ranged from 8.2% in Oregon and 14.6% in Utah to more than 40% in both Pennsylva-nia and Connecticut.
- Average Medicaid payments per elderly recipient ranged from highs of $20,258, $20,000, and $18,901 in Connecticut, New York, and the District of Columbia, respectively, to lows of $2,867, $4,900, and $5,531 in Oregon, California, and Georgia.
- The proportion of total payments for long-term care ranged from 19.0% in New Mexico and 25.3% in Washington to more than 60% in both Connecticut and North Dakota.
- Though institutional care represents the largest proportion of long-term care spending in every state, the relative share of home care varies from lows of 1.1% in Hawaii and 2.6% in Washington to close to 50% in Wyoming and Alaska, respectively.

Medicaid and State Budgets

Excluding revenues received from the federal government and taxes earmarked for special purposes, Medicaid's share of states' general fund expenditures (i.e., deriving from broad-based taxes) grew from 9.0% in 1989 to 10.5% in 1991 and 14.4% in 2000 (National Associa-tion of State Budget Officers, 2001). Having recently eclipsed higher education (12.2%), Medicaid is now only second to elementary and sec-ondary education (35.7%), and exceeds spending for public assistance (2.5%), corrections (7.0%), and transportation (.9%) combined. Only Medicaid and corrections represent a larger share of state spending in 2000 than they did in 1989. Medicaid's share of total expenditures var-ies from state to state, ranging from lows of 7.2% and 8.5% in Kansas and Hawaii, respectively, to highs of 34.5% and 28.7% in New York and Tennessee.

LONG-TERM CARE REFORM POLICY OPTIONS

Merlis (1999) observes, "The states that are currently spending the least on long-term care are the very states expected to see the greatest increase in their elderly populations and presumably, in demand for long-term care services." For these states, he posits a grim choice between raising tax burdens on working-aged adults and limiting access to quality care. One consequence, he suggests, may be increasing pressure to federalize the program. While talk of federalizing Medicaid may indeed be premature, state policymakers continue to rate controlling nursing home and other expenditures toward the top of their long-term care priorities (Murtaugh et al., 1999). Wiener and Stevenson (1997) identify three broad strategies states may use to do so. One is to offset state expenditures by maximizing Medicare long-term care contributions and by relying more on private resources such as long-term care insurance, improved estate recovery, and the prevention of asset transfers. Another is to make the health care delivery system more efficient through managed care and expanded home- and community-based care options. A third, more traditional option is to reduce Medicaid eligibility, services, and reimbursement. While the effects of some of these options are fairly predictable–tightening eligibility and cutting reimbursement lowers expenditures–the efficacy of other strategies for controlling expenditures is more doubtful. Though research evidence indicates that managed care plans serving the elderly operate more cheaply and use fewer resources than traditional fee-for-service arrangements (Brown et al., 1993; Burstein, White, & Kidder, 1996; McCall et al., 1996; Miller, Weissert, & Chernew, 1998), more recent developments in the field of acute and long-term care integration have yet to be fully evaluated (Miller, 2001). Home care also continues to thrive, although it may not be as cost-effective as proponents suggest (Weissert, Cready, & Pawelak, 1988; Weissert & Hedrick, 1994). As with the rest of the Medicaid program, the federal government grants states substantial flexibility in adopting strategies to reform long-term care. Not surprisingly, the combination of strategies and the intensity with which they are pursued vary from state to state.

Maximizing Other Resources:
Offsetting State Contributions with Private Resources

Four states, Connecticut, Indiana, California, and New York, provide higher-level asset protection under Medicaid to individuals who purchase state-approved private long-term care insurance policies (Tilly, Wiener, & Goldenson, 2000). Eighteen states offer tax deductions and credits for purchasers of private long-term care insurance, while another 18 introduced such legislation in 1999. Still another 19 states offer private long-term care insurance benefits to their own employees or retirees.

In 1993, the federal government mandated that states implement estate recovery programs to recover the costs of long-term care and related services from deceased Medicaid recipients. Concomitant with this mandate, the number of states with estate recovery programs grew from 4 in the 1960s, to 14 in the 1980s, and to 45 by the mid-1990s. State policies and procedures on enforcement, however, vary significantly (Sabatino & Wood, 1996).

Delivery System Reform: Managed Care

Through federal waivers of Medicaid program requirements, the number of states enrolling elderly Medicaid recipients in risk-based managed care programs grew from 11 to 25 between 1990 and 1998, while the total number of Medicaid recipients enrolled in such plans increased from 1.5 to 13.5 million (Kaye, Pernice, & Pelletier, 1999). Though most managed care programs for elderly and disabled Medicaid recipients are voluntary and serve limited service areas and enrollments, a small but growing number of states have sought to use managed care as the vehicle for integrating acute and long-term care services for Medicare-Medicaid dual eligibility (Miller, 2001). In addition to Medicaid waivers, many of these latter programs also require Medicare waivers as well. Examples include Minnesota Senior Health Options, the Wisconsin Partnership Program, and MassHealth Senior Care Options. Only the Arizona Long-Term Care System serves both the acute and long-term care needs of this population on a statewide, mandatory basis. While the Balanced Budget Act of 1997 eliminated the need to obtain waivers to enroll most Medicaid populations in mandatory managed care programs, Medicaid recipients dually enrolled with Medicare were among the populations excluded.

Delivery System Reform: Home- and Community-Based Care

Waivers to expand home- and community-based service (HCBS) options to Medicaid recipients who otherwise would have been eligible for Medicaid-funded institutional care have grown as well. While only six states had 1915(c) HCBS waivers in 1982, by 1999, all states but Arizona (which provides long-term care through its 1115 Research and Demonstration waiver) had at least one waiver program, with the total number of Medicaid recipients served increasing from 234,470 to 559,903 between 1992 and 1997 (Lutzky et al., 2000). The number of programs and the particular services and populations covered by each of these programs vary from state to state. Possible services include adult day care, assistive technology, adaptive equipment, case management, personal care attendant, habilitation, homemaker, home health aid, nursing care, personal care, respite care, and caregiver training. States may also seek approval from CMS to cover other services. In addition to 1915(c) waivers, some states have begun to experiment with consumer-directed home care programs for the elderly (Tilly & Wiener, 2001), while 35 other states covered or planned to cover assisted living services through Medicaid (Mollica, 1998). Thirty-two states also report having at least one state-only funded home- and community-based care program (Kassner & Williams, 1997).

Traditional Strategies: Benefits

Federal Medicaid rules require that states provide two mandatory long-term care services, nursing facility services for recipients 21 and over, and home health services for individuals who are entitled to nursing facility care. Because states are free to establish the scope and duration of Medicaid services, however, spending and utilization vary widely. States also have the choice of covering a wide range of optional services and receive federal matching funds for the costs of those benefits, including institutional care for individuals with mental retardation, personal care, and home- and community-based waiver services for individuals who otherwise would be eligible for institutional care. All have chosen to cover intermediate care facilities for the mentally retarded (ICF-MR). Thirty-one states, on the other hand, have chosen to cover personal care services, which include a range of human assistance to persons with disabilities and chronic conditions. Various states have also chosen to cover hospice (38), physical therapy (45), occupational therapy (36), rehabilitation services (53), targeted case management (46), and, of course, 1915(c) HCBS waiver benefits (Committee on Ways and Means, 2000). States wanting to cut back on their Medicaid long-term care commitments have the option of discontinuing coverage of optional services such as these.

Traditional Strategies: Supply of Providers

Regulating the supply of services has been a strategy long used by states interested in controlling long-term care expenditures. States regulate supply, in particular, through certificate of need programs that require nursing homes and other providers to obtain state approval before construction of new facilities or major renovations of old ones. Some also establish moratoriums on new construction altogether or on the certification of new Medicaid beds. In 1998, 38 states had certificate of need programs for nursing facilities, while 19 had implemented moratoriums. Nineteen states, moreover, had enacted certificate of need programs for the formation of home health agencies; one had implemented a moratorium. Some also use certificate of need and moratoriums to control the supply of non-medical residential long-term care facilities as well as the conversion of hospital beds to skilled nursing home beds (Harrington et al., 2000).

Traditional Strategies: Financial and Categorical Eligibility

Medicaid eligibility policy is complex and confusing. Like other aspects of the Medicaid program, there is substantial variation from state to state. As Bruen et al. (1999) observe, "The federal government requires states to cover certain mandatory groups, but states have significant discretion over optional eligibility criteria. . . . Some states provide optional coverage well above the mandatory levels; others provide very little optional coverage." Individuals qualifying for Medicaid must belong to certain categories. One such category is the elderly, defined as individuals aged 65 and older. Being elderly, however, is only a necessary condition for entitlement. To receive benefits, individuals must also qualify financially, which requires that they meet certain income and asset criteria. In most states, individuals who are eligible for Supplemental Security Income (SSI) benefits, the federal welfare program for the aged, blind, and disabled, are also eligible for Medicaid. For individuals, the federal 2001 SSI limit was $531 per month in countable income and no more than $2,000 in assets. The major exceptions to automatic Medicaid coverage for SSI recipients are 11 so called "209(b) states," which are allowed to implement more restrictive eligibility and asset limits, provided that they are not more restrictive than what was used on January 1, 1972. When determining eligibility, the 209(b) states, however, are required to deduct incurred medical expenses from applicants' income.

Federal law also requires states to cover at least a portion of Medicare Part B premiums and/or cost sharing under the Qualified Medicare Beneficiary (QMB), Specified Low-Income Medicare Beneficiary (SLMB), and Qualifying Individuals programs. In 1996, however, close to half of the 5.1 million potentially eligible Medicare beneficiaries did not enroll in either the QMB or SLMB programs (United States General Accounting Office, 1999). Possible reasons include limited program awareness among beneficiaries, a burdensome and complex enrollment process, and limited efforts on the part of states to recruit potential recipients. One study, in particular, found that few states undertook aggressive outreach: only eight used materials in languages other than English; 16 stationed eligibility workers outside welfare offices; 19 used mail or phone applications without face-to-face interviews; 20 received data from CMS identifying low-income Medicare enrollees; and 9 allowed applicants to self-certify the truth of the information contained in their applications (Nemore, 1999).

States also have the option of extending eligibility to other groups. In fact, one study estimates that close to half of Medicaid expenditures are for populations and services that states are not required to cover (Kaiser Commission, 1999). In 1999, for instance, 12 states and the District of Columbia used an option provided by the Omnibus Reconciliation Act of 1986 that allows states to extend Medicaid benefits to aged and disabled individuals with incomes up to 100% of the federal poverty level. That same year as many as 37 states also extended optional Medicaid coverage to individuals with incomes too high to qualify for SSI but who received cash assistance payments known as State Supplemental Payments (Bruen et al., 1999). Under the "300% rule" an additional 34 states provided optional nursing home coverage to individuals with incomes up to 300% of the federal SSI standard ($1,536 per month in 2000) (Kassner & Shirley, 2000). Twenty-nine states, moreover, cover "medically needy" nursing home residents whose incomes exceed the SSI standard but who may "spend down" to Medicaid coverage by incurring medical expenses, which when deducted from their income, brought them below specified eligibility levels. Except for a small personal allowance, institutionalized recipients must contribute most of their income toward the cost of care. In 1998, monthly personal allowances ranged from the $30 minimum in 21 states to 11 states that allowed residents to keep more than $40 per month (Kassner & Shirley, 2000). Protected income and assets for spouses remaining in the community, on the other hand, ranged from $1,357 to $2,019 and $16,152 to $80,760, respectively.

Traditional Strategies: Functional Eligibility

The federal government requires that states perform a comprehensive assessment to determine the functional eligibility of Medicaid nursing home and HCBS waiver applicants. Each state, however, has considerable freedom to sets its own standards (Harrington & Curtis, 1996). Approximately half of all states (24), for example, use "medical/functional" criteria to determine nursing home eligibility, which include the need for nursing services and assessment of cognitive functioning and ability to perform activities of daily living (e.g., bathing, dressing, toileting), while the other half (22) uses "comprehensive" criteria, which include the aforementioned medical/functional standards in addition to an assessment of social factors (e.g., presence of an informal caregiver) and instrumental activities of daily living (e.g., taking medications, financial management) (Snow, 1995). The specific criteria and thresholds used to determine functional eligibility also vary considerably from state to state. Although some consensus exists that nursing needs and physical and cognitive functioning should be considered, there is "no consensus on how these factors should be defined, measured, weighted, and combined to determine minimum functional eligibility criteria" (O'Keefe, 1996). Of 42 states responding to a survey on Medicaid HCBS waiver programs, 6 used scored assessment instruments that require applicants to receive a minimum score in order to achieve eligibility, 19 selected a minimum number of specific impairments or long-term care needs for eligibility requirements to be met, while 17 provided assessors with definitions and general guidelines to guide them through the assessment process (O'Keefe, 1996). A growing number of states have expanded their screening activities to include private pay individuals under the assumption that they would likely exhaust their income and assets and subsequently qualify for Medicaid.

Traditional Strategies: Reimbursement

As with eligibility, services, and other Medicaid system attributes, the federal government has granted states substantial flexibility in setting its own rates and methodologies for reimbursing long-term care providers. In 1997, for example, reimbursement levels for nursing homes varied significantly across states, ranging from a low average per diem of $57 to a high of $237, with an overall cross-state average of $95.09 (Swan et al., 2000). Although 33 states increased their rates in 1997, only 3 had increases greater than 10% after controlling for inflation. Eighteen, on the other hand, witnessed reductions.

Swan and colleagues (2000) categorize states' general reimbursement methodologies as retrospective systems, prospective facility- or patient-specific systems, adjusted systems, combination systems, and flat-rate or prospective-class systems. With retrospective reimbursement, states reimburse nursing homes for the actual costs incurred after care has been delivered. This generally provides facilities with few incentives to achieve economy, perhaps explaining why the number of states relying on purely retrospective reimbursement declined from 13 in 1979 to 1 in 1997 (Swan et al., 2000). With prospective reimbursement, on the other hand, states set rates in advance without subsequent adjustment for full actual costs, placing providers at risk if the cost of providing care exceeds the payments received from Medicaid, and providing them with a profit if payment exceeds their costs. While facility-specific arrangements establish rates based on each individual facility's historical costs, patient-specific systems combine facility-specific costs with a component derived from individual resident attributes. Some, however, use weaker arrangements, including prospective adjusted systems, which establish interim rates that may be adjusted upward though not equal to costs, and combination systems, which retrospectively reimburse for some cost centers while prospectively reimbursing for others. While the number of facility/patient-specific reimbursement systems increased from 17 to 21 between 1979 and 1997, the number of adjusted and combination systems increased from 16 to 32 between 1979 and 1990 before declining to 26 in 1997 (Swan et al., 2000). Unlike these systems, which base their rates on the costs of each individual facility, prospective-class or flat-rate systems establish the same rate for all facilities within a specified group. Between 1979 and 1997, the number of states with flat-rate systems remained steady at around three or four per year (Swan et al., 2000).

Besides their general methodology, states make several other choices when establishing their reimbursement policies (Holahan, 1985). For example, states must determine whether and how homes should be grouped for purposes of establishing ceilings (e.g., by size, ownership, or region). They must also determine whether total costs or individual cost centers (e.g., nursing, administration, profits, capital, room and board) should have ceiling limitations and whether the percentile ceilings on allowable costs should be set high or low. Other issues include what kind of inflation allowances should be used in projecting targets in prospective systems, and in setting interim rates in retrospective systems, and whether efficiency bonuses should be employed. What ancillaries, if any, should be included in their rates (e.g., physical therapy, occupational therapy, prescription drugs, medical supplies, durable medical equipment), and how property costs should be valued are also issues states must consider. A growing number of states also employ case mix methods to counteract access problems for heavy care patients and to distribute payment more equitably across providers. Between 1979 and 1997, in particular, the number of states adjusting for case mix increased from 3 to 26 (Swan et al., 2000).

MEDICAID OVER THE LAST TWENTY YEARS

Because the federal government grants states significant flexibility in Medicaid program administration, there is tremendous cross-state variation in expenditures and populations served. This variation is also evident in the various long-term care reform strategies pursued by state governments. These include offsetting state contributions with private resources, adding managed care and home- and community-based care services options, in addition to relying on a variety of more traditional strategies related to available benefits, providers, eligibility, and reimbursement. Though a substantial level of discretion has always existed, its extent has varied over the course of the program's development. Compared to the first decade and a half of the program's existence, in particular, the last 20 years have represented an especially active period of intergovernmental give-and-take, in which proposals to reform Medicaid policy have hinged on various views regarding the proper balance of power between the national and state governments, and whether greater responsibility for program functions should be devolved to the states. Prior to 1980, in particular, there was comparatively little federal intrusion into the way states ran their Medicaid programs. After 1981, however, federal efforts to shape the program grew. Between 1965 and 1983, for example, Gilman (1998) recorded 27 significant changes in program eligibility, benefits, and funding, including five major eligibility expansions, only one of which was mandatory. Between 1984 and 1990, however, Gilman recorded 54 changes, including 19 mandatory eligibility expansions and 12 optional expansions.

Though states had initially supported some of these expansions, recession and double-digit increases in program expenditures quickly led most to seek an end to new mandates. In the meantime, however, states increasingly took advantage of a loophole in the Medicaid law that enabled them to use provider tax and donation schemes, which in combination with disproportionate share hospital (DSH) payments, allowed them to draw billions of federal matching funds into their treasuries with little, if any, additional state outlays (Coughlin, Ku, & Holahan, 1994). "Just as the states cried 'foul' when confronted with mandated expansions," federal officials "decried tax-DSH arrangements as 'scams,' 'gimmicks,' 'con games,' and worse" (Hegner, 1997). The federal government effectively put a halt to this practice with the Medicaid Voluntary Contributions and Provider-Specific Tax Amendments of 1991. At the same time, changes in the congressional budget process made it more difficult for advocates to push through Medicaid expansions by forcing them to be explicit about the long-term costs of such extensions. Particular changes included making budget figures binding for three years rather than one year, and requiring that any new extensions be tied to proportionate adjustments in revenues or cuts in other programs (Gilman, 1998).

Though these changes helped end the adoption of mandatory program expansions after 1990, President Clinton and the Republican Congress worked together to pass the 1995 Unfunded Mandates Reform Act, which limited the federal government's authority to adopt future mandates for state and local governments without paying for them. The Administration also worked with the Republican majority to pass the Balanced Budget Act (BBA) of 1997, which evolved out of various proposals to restructure Medicaid during the 1995-96 budget debate. The Congressional majority's MediGrant proposal would have eliminated Medicaid's open-ended entitlement and replaced it with a block grant to the states, which would have granted states virtually complete autonomy with respect to payment policy, service delivery, and coverage, and would have eliminated most federal oversight of OBRA 1987's nursing home quality standards. The administration, on the other hand, advocated enhanced budgetary control and expanded state discretion but kept Medicaid's basic structure intact. Viewing Medicaid reform as a way to gain control of the fastest growing portion of their budgets, the National Governor's Association proposed combining elements of Congress' block grant approach with a per beneficiary limit on expenditure growth proposed by the President (Feder, Lambrew, & Huckaby, 1996).

In the end, the President's incremental approach won out, in part, because of concerns about nursing home quality associated with the majority's block grant proposal. In addition to repealing the Boren Amendment, which nursing facilities and other providers had used to sue states over reimbursement, the BBA gave states the option of enrolling most Medicaid beneficiaries in managed care programs without seeking waivers (a process the administration had already accelerated), while giving them substantially more freedom in choosing the types of plans with which they contracted. The BBA also made the Program for All-Inclusive Care of the Elderly permanent under Medicare and a state option under Medicaid, and created the State Children's Health Insurance Program (SCHIP), which offers federal matching funds for states and territories that provide health insurance coverage to uninsured, low-income children.

At the extreme, then, devolution implied federal government withdrawal from funding health care for the poor (DiIulio & Nathan, 1998). Though no proposals suggested such a radical step, the Republicans' desire to shift Medicaid from an open-ended entitlement to a block grant would have come close. The result, instead, was the incremental approach of the BBA, which provided for a variety of changes at the program's margins that enhanced state discretion in areas such as provider payment and managed care. Comparatively restrained changes such as these should not be dismissed, however, as the accumulation of incremental changes can have broad implications for the balance of intergovernmental power (DiIulio & Nathan, 1998).

MEDICAID AND DEVOLUTION

To a large extent, the debate over devolution that has framed recent Medicaid history revolves around varying assessments of the administrative and fiscal capacities of the states to assume the burdens and opportunities that devolution would entail. It also revolves around varying assessments of the types of policy commitments likely to bubble up from state political processes as compared to those at the national level. Would states be willing, for example, to fund health insurance programs for low-income individuals? Or, for example, could states, in the absence of federal guidelines, be trusted to develop and implement reimbursement methods that sufficiently balanced the goal of cost containment with concerns about quality, access, and equitable provider payment? Proponents of devolution, on the one hand, seek to enlarge state power over Medicaid. According to Tallon and Brown (1998), "(e)nthusiasm for Medicaid devolution draws strength from growing skepticism about the wisdom of federal policy rules, increased confidence in the capacities of the states, declining legitimacy of the poor (and of social programs that assist them), state resentment over federal mandates, and mounting federal irritation over state 'scams' to attract extra federal funds." In the area of long-term care, in particular, proponents suggest that granting state discretion would better allow them to take advantage of their considerable experience in managing day-to-day program operations, including assessing client needs, regulating supply, processing claims, coordinating care, and setting reimbursement rates. Since long-term care is such a highly personal service, moreover, they argue that planning and delivery should be influenced by local norms, circumstances, and values, and by local preferences of the recipients, their caregivers, and providers (Wiener, 1998). More generally, devolution advocates assert that state and locally administered programs are less rigid and bureaucratic than nationally run programs. They also point out that "federal officials cannot anticipate every eventuality" and that "state and local conditions vary in ways that affect the selection of an optimal strategy to achieve goals" (Davidson, 1997). The role of states as policy innovators and the freedom from federal rules they need in order to experiment is another reason frequently highlighted.

Those in favor of a stronger federal role, on the other hand, fear a race-to-the-bottom dynamic if national standards are loosened or lifted (Peterson, 1995). Since the federal government pays more than half of Medicaid program costs, moreover, they argue that states need to be held accountable for how that money is spent. They also believe that it is the job of the national government to reduce, or bring within an acceptable range, any undesirable variation that arises from varying state commitments and willingness to act. Recognizing that states have their own political, economic, social and cultural histories, they argue that in a federal system, it is the national government's role to promote equity across geographic regions, where the accident of one's birth or residency should not influence one's ability to obtain health care. Proponents also want to avoid the negative effects that widely differing social conditions might entail for the common foundations on which society and government rest (Davidson, 1997).

But how much variation is too much and how much variation is too little? The answer depends on one's views regarding the advantages and disadvantages of greater or lesser state control. On the one hand, proponents of devolution view state Medicaid variation favorably. They see it as reflecting state control over a policy area in which local preferences should predominate. Opponents, on the other hand, view it unfavorably. To them, it reflects abandonment of federal responsibility for ensuring equity in the distribution of health and long-term care financing and services. Regardless of one's position, however, there can be little doubt that substantial state discretion already exists, as evidenced by the tremendous amount of cross-state variation documented here.

CONCLUSION

Because of substantial flexibility granted states in administering Medicaid, there are essentially 56 separate programs covering each of the 50 states, territories, and the District of Columbia. This is one reason why there is so much variability in Medicaid program characteristics around the country, not only in terms of program coverage and expenditures but also in terms of available strategies to reform the delivery and financing of long-term care. It would seem, then, that most responsibility for caring for the poor and disabled elderly has already been devolved to the states. Since there is little doubt that states take full advantage of the discretion afforded by this arrangement, advocates of devolution may want to reassess their views to consider whether existing variation has resulted in inequities addressable only through more, not less, federal involvement.

AUTHOR NOTES

Edward Alan Miller received his AB and MPA from Cornell University and his MA in political science from the University of Michigan. He is currently a doctoral candidate in political science and health services organization and policy. Prior to his studies, he worked as a health policy researcher and writer and studied in New Zealand as a Fulbright Scholar. His current research interests include long-term care, managed care, organization theory, and intergovernmental relations. His dissertation seeks to understand state adoption of changes in Medicaid nursing facility reimbursement methods and rates over time.

Mr. Miller can be contacted at the Department of Health Management & Policy, School of Public Health, The University of Michigan, 109 S. Observatory, Ann Arbor, MI 48109 (E-mail: eddiemil@umich.edu).

REFERENCES

Brown, R. S., Clement, G. G., & Hill, J. W. (1993). Do health maintenance organizations work for Medicare? *Health Care Financing Review, 15,* 7-23.

Bruen, B., & Holahan, J. (1999). *Slow Growth in Medicaid Spending Continues in 1997.* Washington, DC: Kaiser Commission on Medicaid and the Uninsured.

Bruen, B. K., Wiener, J. M., Kim, J., & Miazad, O. (1999). *State usage of Medicaid Coverage Options for Aged, Blind, and Disabled People. Assessing the New Federalism.* Washington, DC: The Urban Institute.

Burstein, N. R., White, A. J., & Kidder, D. (1996). *Evaluation of the Program of All-Inclusive Care for the Elderly (PACE) Demonstration: The Impact of PACE on Outcomes.* Cambridge, Massachusetts: Abt Associations.

Burwell, B. (2001). *Medicaid Long-Term Care Expenditures in FY 2000.* Cambridge, Massachusetts: The MEDSTAT Group.

Centers for Medicare and Medicaid Services (CMS), U. S. Department of Health and Human Services. (2002a). *Medicaid Financial Statistics (HCFA-64 Report).* Baltimore, Maryland: CMS, USDHHS.

Centers for Medicare and Medicaid Services (CMS), U. S. Department of Health and Human Services (2002b). *Medicaid Program Statistics (HCFA-2082 Report). http://www.hcfa.gov/medicaid/msis/mstats.htm.* Site Visited 1/15/02. Baltimore, Maryland: CMS, USDHHS.

Committee on Ways and Means, U.S. House of Representatives (2000, October 6). *2000 Greenbook: Background Material and Data on Programs Within the Jurisdiction of the Committee on Ways and Means.* 106-14.

Congressional Budget Office (CBO) (1997). *CBO Memorandum, Budgetary Implications of the Balanced Budget Act of 1997.* Washington, DC: CBO.

Congressional Budget Office (CBO) (1999). *CBO Memorandum, Projections of Expenditures for Long-Term Care Services for the Elderly.* Washington, DC: CBO.

Coughlin, T. A., Ku, L., & Holahan, J. (1994). *Medicaid Since 1980: Costs, Coverage, and the Shifting Alliance Between the Federal Government and the States.* Washington, DC: The Urban Institute Press.

Davidson, S. M. (1997). Politics matters! Health care policy and the federal system. *Journal of Health Politics, Policy, and Law, 22*(3), 879-896.

DiIulio, Jr., J. J., & Nathan, R. P. (1998). Introduction. In F. J. Thompson and J. J. DiIulio (Eds.), *Medicaid and Devolution: A View from the States* (pp. 1-13). Washington, DC: Brookings Institution Press.

Feder, J., Lambrew, J., & Huckaby, M. (1996). *Medicaid and Long-Term Care for the Elderly.* New York, New York: The Commonwealth Fund.

Gilman, J. D. (1998). Medicaid and the costs of federalism, 1984-1992. In J. G. Bruhn (Ed.), *Health Care Policy in the United States.* New York: Garland Publishing, Inc.

Harrington, C., & Curtis, M. (1996). State variations and trends in preadmission screening programs. *The Journal of Applied Gerontology, 15*(4), 414-432.

Harrington, C., Swan, J. H., Wellin, V., Clemena, W., & Carrillo, H. M. (2000). *1998 State Data Book on Long-Term Care Program and Market Characteristics.* San Francisco, CA: Department of Social and Behavioral Sciences.

Health Care Financing Administration (HCFA), U. S. Department of Health and Human Services (2000). *Personal Health Care Expenditures.* Baltimore, Maryland: HCFA, USDHHS.

Hegner, R. E. (1997). *Intergovernmental Relations in American Health Policy: Potential Partnership or Perpetual Tug of War.* Washington, DC: National Health Policy Forum, Technical Advisory Committee on Devolution and Federalism.

Holahan, J. (1985). State rate-setting and its effects on the cost of nursing-home care. *Journal of Health Politics, Policy, and Law, 9*(4), 647-667.

Holahan, J., & Liska, D. (1998). Variations in Medicaid spending among the states. Vol. No. A-3, *Assessing the New Federalism, Series A*. Washington, DC: The Urban Institute.

Kaiser Commission on Medicaid and the Uninsured (1999). *Medicaid: A Primer, An Introduction and Overview*. Washington, DC: The Henry J. Kaiser Family Foundation.

Kassner, E., & Shirley, L. (2000). *Medicaid Financial Eligibility for Older People: State Variations in Access to Home and Community-Based Waiver and Nursing Home Services*. Washington, DC: AARP, Public Policy Institute.

Kassner, E., & Williams, L. (1997). *Taking Care of Their Own: State-Funded Home and Community-Based Care Programs for Older Persons*. Washington, DC: AARP, Public Policy Institute.

Kaye, N., Pernice, C., & Pelletier, H. (1999). *Medicaid Managed Care: A Guide for States*, Fourth Edition. Portland, Maine: National Academy for State Health Policy.

Lutzky, S, Alecxih, L. M. B., Duffy, J., & Neill, C. (2000). *Review of the Medicaid 1915(c) and Community-Based Services Waiver Program Literature and Program Data: Final Report*. Prepared for the Department of Health and Human Services, Health Care Financing Administration. Contract No. 500-96-0005. The Lewin Group, Inc.

McCall, N. et al. (1996). *Evaluation of Arizona's Health Care Cost Containment System Demonstration*. Final Report. San Francisco, California: Laguna Research Associates.

Merlis, M. (1999). *Financing Long-Term Care in the Twenty-First Century: The Public and Private Roles*. New York: The Commonwealth Fund.

Miller, E. A. (2001). *Federal and State Initiatives to Integrate Acute and Long-Term Care: Issues and Profiles*. RL30813. Washington, DC: Congressional Research Services.

Miller, E. A., Weissert, W. G., & Chernew, M. (1998). Managed care for the elderly people: A compendium of findings. *American Journal of Medical Quality, 13*(3), 127-140.

Mollica, R. L. (1998). *State Assisted Living Policy, 1998*. August, Maine: National Academy for State Health Policy.

Murtaugh, C., Sparer, M. S., Feldman, P. H., Lee, J. S., Basch, A., Sherlock, A., & Clark, A. L. (1999). *State Strategies for Allocating Resources to Home- and Community-Based Care*. New York: Center for Home Care Policy and Research, Visiting Nurse Services of New York.

National Association of State Budget Officers (NASBO). (2001). *2000 State Expenditure Report*. Washington, DC: National Association of State Budget Officers.

Nemore, P. B. (1999). *Variations in State Medicaid Buy-In Practices for Low-Income Medicare Beneficiaries: A 1999 Update*. Washington, DC: National Senior Citizens Law Center.

Niefield, M., O'Brien, E., & Feder, J. (1999). *Long-Term Care: Medicaid's Role and Challenges*. Washington, DC: Henry J. Kaiser Foundation.

O'Keefe, J. (1996). *Determining the Need for Long-Term Care Services: An Analysis of Health and Functional Eligibility Criteria in Medicaid Home- and Community-Based Waiver Programs*. Washington, DC: AARP.

Peterson, P. E. (1995). *The Price of Federalism*. Washington, DC: The Brookings Institution.

Sabatino, C. P., & Wood, E. (1996). *Medicaid Estate Recovery: A Survey of State Programs and Practices*. Washington, DC: AARP, Public Policy Institute.

Snow, K. I. (1995). *How States Determine Nursing Facility Eligibility for the Elderly: A National Survey.* Washington, DC: AARP, Public Policy Institute.

Swan, J. H., Harrington, C., Clemena, W., Struder, L., & de Wit, S. K. (2000). Medicaid nursing facility reimbursement methods: 1979-1997. *Medical Care Research and Review, 57*(3), 361-378.

Tallon, J. R., & Brown, L. D. (1998). Who gets what? Devolution of eligibility and benefits in Medicaid. In F. J. Thompson and J. J. DiIulio (Eds.), *Medicaid and Devolution: A View from the States* (pp. 235-257). Washington, DC: Brookings Institution Press.

The Lewin Group, Inc. (2000). *The Long-Term Care Financing Model.* Prepared by The Lewin Group, Inc. for the Department of Health and Human Services.

Thompson, F. J. (1998). The faces of devolution. In F. J. Thompson and J. J. DiIulio (Eds.), *Medicaid and Devolution: A View from the States* (pp. 14-55). Washington, DC: Brookings Institution Press.

Tilly, J., & Wiener, J. M. (2001). Consumer-Directed Home and Community Services: Policy Issues. Occasional Paper, Number 44. Washington, DC: The Urban Institute.

Tilly, J., Wiener, J. M., & Goldenson, S. M. (2000). Federal and state initiatives to jump start the market for private long-term care insurance. *The Elder Law Journal, 8*, 57-102.

United States General Accounting Office (USGAO). (1999). *Low-Income Medicare Beneficiaries: Further Outreach and Administrative Simplification Could Increase Enrollment.* Washington, DC: United States General Accounting Office.

Weissert, W. G., Cready, C. M., & Pawelak, J. E. (1988). The past and future of home- and community-based long-term care. *Milbank Memorial Fund Quarterly, 66*, 309-388.

Weissert, W. G., & Hedrick, S. C. (1994). Lessons learned from research on effects of community-based long-term care. *Journal of the American Geriatrics Society, 42*, 348-353.

Wiener, J. M. (1998). Long-term care and devolution. In F. J. Thompson and J. J. DiIulio (Eds.), *Medicaid and Devolution: A View from the States* (pp. 185-234). Washington, DC: Brookings Institution Press.

Wiener, J. M., & Stevenson, D.G. (1997). *Long-Term Care for the Elderly and State Health Policy.* Vol. No. A-17, *New Federalism: Issues and Options for States, Series A.* Washington, DC: The Urban Institute.

Wiener, J. M., Tilly, J., & Goldenson, S. M. (2000). Federal and state initiatives to jump-start the market for private long-term care insurance. *Elder Law Journal, 8*(11), 57-99.

Devolution of Employment and Training Policy: The Case of Older Workers

Peter Doeringer, PhD

Boston University

Andrew Sum, PhD

Northeastern University

David Terkla, PhD

University of Massachusetts Boston

SUMMARY. The case for the devolution of employment and training programs has traditionally been based on the supply side argument that state and local governments are in the best position to assess the training needs of their disadvantaged workers. We provide a different perspective by focusing on the demand side of the labor market and the link between aiding older workers and fostering economic growth. We illustrate the importance of this focus by examining the labor market in Massachusetts, where the full employment economy of the late 1990s resulted in serious labor supply bottlenecks. Older workers, whose ranks are growing rapidly, provide the largest known labor reserve for meeting these labor supply deficits in the next decade. Tapping this reserve, however, means improving skills, deferring retirement, bringing older persons back into the labor market, and increasing full-time employment.

Massachusetts already has the policy tools needed to train older workers to fill emerging job needs, but these policies will need to be substantially up-

[Haworth co-indexing entry note]: "Devolution of Employment and Training Policy: The Case of Older Workers." Doeringer, Peter, Andrew Sum, and David Terkla. Co-published simultaneously in *Journal of Aging & Social Policy* (The Haworth Press, Inc.) Vol. 14, No. 3/4, 2002, pp. 37-60; and: *Devolution and Aging Policy* (ed: Francis G. Caro, and Robert Morris) The Haworth Press, Inc., 2002, pp. 37-60. Single or multiple copies of this article are available for a fee from The Haworth Document Delivery Service [1-800-HAWORTH, 9:00 a.m. - 5:00 p.m. (EST). E-mail address: getinfo@haworthpressinc.com].

10.1300/J031v14n03_03

graded and reoriented. Too little funding, an emphasis on short-term programs, lack of coordination among programs, weak linkages to the private sector, and the limited flexibility of human resources practices in both the private and public sectors have left both government programs and employers ill-prepared to utilize fully the older worker labor reserve. *[Article copies available for a fee from The Haworth Document Delivery Service: 1-800-HAWORTH. E-mail address: <getinfo@haworthpressinc.com> Website: <http://www.HaworthPress.com> © 2002 by The Haworth Press, Inc. All rights reserved.]*

KEYWORDS. Older workers, training programs, full employment, labor scarcities, labor reserves

INTRODUCTION

The general case for the devolution of employment and training programs has traditionally been based on the argument that state and local governments are in a better position than the federal government to assess and plan for meeting the training needs of local groups of unemployed, displaced, and disadvantaged workers. Critics of devolution, however, maintain that a strong federal presence is needed to ensure that resources are allocated equitably among those most in need and that program quality is maintained. While there is little evidence to support either side of this debate, the last few decades have seen a sharp reduction in federal influence over employment and training programs.

This paper provides a different perspective on the devolution of employment and training policy by looking at the demand side of the labor market and at the link between the goal of aiding the unemployed, displaced, and disadvantaged workers and the goal of fostering economic growth. Rapid job growth and the full employment economy of the late 1990s resulted in serious labor supply bottlenecks that could best be addressed through training programs targeted on skill scarcities and the upgrading of employed and underemployed workers. Since the composition of skill scarcities varies considerably from state to state, and even from employer to employer within states, we argue that a focus on economic growth strengthens the case for a decentralized employment and training system that can be targeted at local skill needs. We stress, however, that the effectiveness of such a decentralized system depends on having stronger performance assessments and a greater emphasis on wage and skill upgrading than has previously been the case.

We illustrate the importance of reorienting state and local employment and training policy towards skill upgrading and economic development by examining the labor market for older workers. Changes in the demographics of the U.S. working-age population will make older workers (45-64) the primary source of labor for meeting skill scarcities over the next decade. However, tapping this older worker resource to eliminate skill bottlenecks in high growth sectors will require substantial adjustments in workplace human resources practices, as well as far more substantial investments in the training of older workers, than has occurred in the past.

THE DEVOLUTION IN EMPLOYMENT AND TRAINING POLICY

U.S. employment and training policies in the post-war period began in the early 1960s under the initiative and control of the federal government, but subsequently experienced the same pressures for the "new federalism" as most other social welfare programs. Today, the governance of federally funded employment and training programs is almost exclusively the responsibility of state and local employment and training agencies under the Workforce Investment Act of 1998 (WIA). This extensive devolution of responsibility from the federal government to state and local governments, however, has followed a more erratic path than that of many other social programs.

The first manpower programs of the post-World War era, the Area Redevelopment Act of 1961 and the Manpower Development and Training Act of 1962, grew out of concerns with structural imbalances in the economy (Mangum et al., 1998). Unlike the WPA, CCC, and other New Deal programs that focused on job creation as the solution to unemployment, these programs largely concentrated on preparing the unemployed for existing jobs.

The earliest programs were essentially demonstration efforts directed at a selected group of labor markets characterized by structural change and industrial dislocation. The design, implementation, and evaluation of most of these programs were centrally administered by the U.S. Department of Labor. Often, these programs worked in conjunction with the federal-state employment services system, which had a national network of state and local offices, and there were various other informal sources of state and local input.

By the mid-1960s, however, training programs began to proliferate, funding levels increased, and the emphasis of employment and training policy shifted from structural unemployment to poverty. Job creation programs such as the Neighborhood Youth Corps, the Work Experience Program, New Careers, and Operation Mainstream were added to the policy mix to provide new employment opportunities for youth, adult welfare recipients, and older workers.

In response to the growing size and complexity of manpower programs, the federal government tried a series of different approaches for linking federal resources to state and local labor market needs (Mucciaroni, 1990). The first step towards a closer relationship with state and local labor markets kept program governance in the hands of the federal government, but moved program responsibility from Washington to the regional offices of the U.S. Labor Department. By 1968, this regional approach to federal control of manpower policy was augmented with a new planning and coordination system known as the Cooperative Area Manpower Planning System (CAMPS), which gave states and local areas formal input into federal policies in their regions.

The next step in this devolution was to shift program governance to state and local governments by giving states and large cities what amounted to categorical block grants for training and subsidized public sector employment under the Comprehensive Employment and Training Act of 1973 (CETA). CETA was initially subject only to broad federal oversight, but the lack of a consistent nationwide focus on the poor led to a reassertion of some federal control in 1978 through federally mandated target populations to be served and by the adoption of federally-determined program performance standards.

This "regulated" decentralization was retained until 1982, when the Job Training Partnership Act (JTPA) replaced CETA. The JTPA reinstituted much of the original CETA structure of block grants under the philosophy of the "New Federalism." However, this new legislation eliminated public job creation as a permissible program activity and it retained separate funding streams and set-asides to ensure dedicated funding allocations for youth and dislocated workers, and for older workers who had traditionally been an underserved population.

The WIA, which replaces JTPA, further extends decentralization by allowing states more flexibility in the use of funds and even more strongly encouraging cooperation among state and local human resources programs. One consequence of this flexibility, however, is that the specially earmarked funding for older workers was eliminated.[1]

What has remained remarkably constant, regardless of which formal structures of governance are in place, is the level of program effectiveness. Program evaluations have routinely confirmed, as recently as the mid-1990s, that adult workers trained through these programs earn modestly more on average than comparable workers without training. They also show that longer training programs yield more earnings improvement than short ones, that employer-based skill programs tend to do better than general classroom training, and that programs for adults are usually more successful than those for youth (Orr et al., 1996; Schochet et al., 2000).[2]

With a few exceptions, such as the Job Corps, these programs have also suffered from a common set of liabilities (Schochet et al., 2000). The programmatic emphasis frequently has been on immediate job placements, rather than on making the kinds of long-term training investments that would upgrade skills and earnings. Classroom training has been favored over developing employer-based training programs, and only nominal attention has been paid to skill scarcities (Mangum, Mangum, & Sum, 1998). As a result, they have largely served the low-skilled end of the job market, and annual earnings improvements have come more often from working longer hours than from higher wages. Furthermore, despite repeated attempts to promote cooperation and coordination among closely related employment and training programs at the state and local levels, program autonomy remains the rule. None of the different versions of decentralization has made much headway in integrating employment and training programs with other programs, such as adult basic education, occupational training by community colleges, and "welfare to work," which have overlapping clienteles and objectives.

It is tempting to trace these persistent flaws in employment and training programs to the continuous devolution of program responsibility from federal to state and local governments. For example, devolution might have allowed state and local governments to avoid the hard challenges of running effective programs, or it might have lodged planning and information gathering at the wrong level of government. However, these are longstanding problems whose solutions have eluded government at all levels.

Instead, the fault lies with a common tendency of government at all levels to spread limited employment and training resources too thinly by focusing on strategies of low-cost placement and short-term training. Careful evaluation of long-term program performance has been neglected by most state and local delivery agents because of the lack of insistence on long-term performance measurement at the federal level and an unwillingness to invest substantial resources in analyses and evaluations that might reveal program shortcomings. Similarly, bureaucratic territoriality has been allowed to dominate meaningful program coordination both at the federal level and at the state and local levels. Overall, there has been too little appreciation of what it takes to train workers for better jobs and too little will to assess performance or undertake the types of reform that might expose underlying program weaknesses.

Because WIA was implemented near the end of a long period of prosperity, there was some prospect that its lofty aims of broadening the range of services available and improving coordination might be achieved. The full employment economy demonstrated that the goal of placing most enrollees in jobs could easily be met. At the same time, full employment generated new political constituencies for employment and training policy in state government and among employers by showing that prosperity and continued growth are vulnerable to problems of unmet labor scarcities. The urgency of filling skilled jobs could have encouraged state and local governments to reorient their planning goals from achieving "work readiness" to meeting labor shortages and promoting wage upgrading.

Substantially raising the wages of the poor or reducing the wage losses of displaced workers continued to prove difficult, even when jobs were plentiful. Nevertheless, the kind of agile and tightly coordinated planning and delivery system envisioned by WIA had the potential for pairing knowledge of local labor markets and employer skill needs with a long-term human resources development program (Mangum, Mangum, & Sum, 1998; LaLonde et al., 2001). The 2002 recession has eroded this potential and at least temporarily closed the window of opportunity for reform. What remain important, however, are the policy lessons for the future provided by the structural changes of the full employment economy of the 1990s.

FULL EMPLOYMENT, LABOR RESERVES, AND OLDER WORKERS

Full employment means that nearly all workers who want jobs are employed. If full employment economies are to continue to grow, underutilized labor reserves must be found to relieve labor supply constraints on growth. During the last decade, the most readily available labor reserves have already been tapped. Female labor force participation rates, which rose rapidly through the early 1990s and are now among the highest in the world, are unlikely to grow much more. Teenage workers continue to have relatively high unemployment rates, but teenagers represent only a temporary labor reserve since their employment rates rise rapidly as they move into their mid-twenties. Legal immigration, which has been a major source of workforce growth in the last decade (especially in Massachusetts and the Northeast region), is subject to quotas that are unlikely to be allowed to rise sufficiently to meet our labor needs and may even fall in the aftermath of national security concerns following the September 11 terrorist attacks. The only remaining labor reserve of sufficient size and certainty to overcome supply constraints on growth is the older workforce (45-69 years old).[3]

The graying of the baby boom generation will mean that the number of older persons (45-69 year olds) in the United States is likely to rise by 46% (28.8 million persons) between 1995 and 2010, nearly three times faster than the rate of growth of the entire working-age population (U.S. Census Bureau, Population Projections to 2050, 2000). As a result, the older worker population will increase its share of the working-age population from slightly below 31% in 1995 to an historic high of almost 40% by 2010. How this demographic shift will affect the nation's civilian labor force in the coming decade depends critically on the labor force participation behavior of older men and women.

Over the past 30 years, there has been a decline in the labor force participation rates of older men (45-64) in the United States (Table 1). In 1999, the labor force participation rate of men 45-54 years old was nearly four percentage points below its 1970 value, while the participation rate of men 55-69 years old was 10-13 percentage points below that prevailing in 1970. This decline in the labor force attachment of older males over the past two decades is disproportionately concentrated among those with the least education (Table 2) who have experienced a reduced demand for their labor and falling real wages. Older dislocated workers with limited schooling face particularly bleak employment prospects and have shown the greatest tendency to withdraw from the labor force (Doeringer et al., 1991).

In contrast to the labor force behavior of older men, older women have substantially increased their attachment to the labor force over the past 30 years (Table 1). These gains accelerated during the 1990s, reflecting a combination of more education and more work experience among the newer cohorts of older women along with rising real wages. Labor force participation rates for older women continue to remain below those of older men, although the size of this gap has narrowed considerably in recent decades.

These secular trends in the participation behavior of older workers are expected to continue over the decade 1998-2008. The U.S. Bureau of Labor Statistics estimates that the labor force participation rate of 45-54-year-old males will be basically unchanged (a decline of 0.4 percentage points), while there will be a modest increase for men in the 55-64 age group (Table 3). Much larger increases in labor force participation rates are projected for older women, with particularly strong gains for women in the 45-54 and 55-64 age groups. Modest growth during the decade will also occur in the labor force participation rates of both men and women in the 65-74-year-old age bracket, as the 54-64-year-old cohort ages. As a consequence of the very high growth rates in the size of the older worker population and the projected increases in their labor force participation rates, older workers will account for nearly all of the growth in the nation's civilian labor force, barring unanticipated increases in foreign immigration.

CHARACTERISTICS OF THE OLDER WORKER LABOR RESERVE

Older workers already contribute substantially to the economy, especially those with high levels of work experience and formal schooling, and on average have lower unemployment rates than younger workers.[4]

TABLE 1. Trends in the Civilian Labor Force Participation Rates of 45-54, 55-64, and 65-69-Year-Old Men and Women, U.S.: Selected Years, 1970 to 1999 (In Percent)

	Age Group					
	(A) 45-54		(B) 55-64		(C) 65-69	
Year	Men	Women	Men	Women	Men	Women
1970	92.4	52.5	80.5	42.0	38.9	17.2
1979	91.4	58.4	73.0	41.9	29.6	15.3
1989	91.1	70.5	67.2	45.0	26.1	16.4
1992	90.8	72.7	67.0	46.6	25.9	16.2
1997	89.5	76.0	67.6	50.9	28.4	17.6
1999	88.8	76.7	67.9	51.5	28.5	18.4
Change, 1970-99	−3.6	+24.2	−12.6	+9.5	−10.4	+1.2
Change, 1989-99	−2.3	+6.2	+.7	+6.5	+2.4	+2.0

Sources: 1970 Census of Population and Housing; U.S. Bureau of Labor Statistics, Employment and Earnings, January 1980, January 1990, January 1993, January 1998, and January 2000.

TABLE 2. Percent of the Older Worker Population in the Civilian Labor Force at Various Ages, Total and by Gender and Educational Attainment: 1998-99 U.S. Averages

	(A)	(B)	(C)	(D)	(E)	(F)	(G)
Age	All	Men	Women	< 12 Years	12 Years	13-15 Years	16 or More
45	85.3	92.0	79.0	70.2	82.9	87.7	91.5
50	82.4	88.9	76.2	62.8	78.3	85.5	90.7
55	74.7	82.7	67.0	56.2	73.0	77.7	84.5
60	58.1	68.3	49.0	44.2	56.3	62.2	71.0
62	45.8	53.5	38.7	30.2	44.3	50.5	61.3
64	34.7	41.2	29.0	25.4	32.4	38.7	46.7
65	29.2	35.8	23.4	20.9	26.4	32.3	42.6
70	16.1	21.0	12.2	12.3	14.5	18.3	24.6

Source: January 1998 to December 1999 CPS public use tapes, tabulations by Center for Labor Market Studies, Northeastern University.

However, the most readily available labor reserves of older workers are those with relatively little education, limited literacy, and a history of job displacement. These older workers routinely experience a variety of labor market problems, including long and repeated spells of unemployment, chronic underemployment, hidden unemployment, and low earnings.[5]

Unemployment among older workers, while below the national average, tends to be of long duration. For example, despite seven years of strong job growth, unemployed older workers in 1999 averaged 17 to 20 weeks of unemployment compared to 9 to 11 weeks among younger unemployed workers. Similarly, a recent survey of dislocated workers found that only 56% of older workers displaced from their jobs over the prior three years (1997-99) had been able to obtain replacement jobs, compared to 80% reemployment rates for younger displaced workers aged 25-54 (U.S. Bureau of Labor Statistics, 2000).

A second labor reserve consists of the "hidden unemployed"–persons who want to be employed, but are not actively looking for work.[6] The estimated average number of older persons (45+) who were among the hidden unemployed each month was 1.3 million or 3% of all older persons (45+) who were not actively participating in the civilian labor force in 1998 and 1999.[7] Such hidden unemployment is particularly a problem among older, displaced workers. The latest national dislocated

TABLE 3. Projected Trends in the Civilian Labor Force Participation Rates of Older Men and Women in Selected Age Groups, U.S.: 1998 to 2008 (Numbers in Percent)

Gender/Age Group	(A) 1998	(B) 2008	(C) Percentage Point Change, 1998-2008
Men			
• 45-54	89.2	88.8	−.4
• 55-64	68.1	69.4	+1.3
• 65-74	22.6	25.5	+2.9
Women			
• 45-54	76.2	80.0	+3.8
• 55-64	51.2	57.7	+6.5
• 65-74	13.7	14.8	+1.1

Source: Fullerton, 1999.

worker survey shows that 30% of displaced older workers (55-64 years old) had withdrawn from the labor force, a rate three times that for those 25-54 years of age.

A third reserve consists of those who are involuntarily working part-time. Approximately 16% of employed 45-69 year old males and 31% of employed older females work part-time, a fraction that has increased steadily since the early 1970s.[8] While a substantial majority of the older part-time employed report that they are working part-time out of personal choice, between 6 and 8% of the part-time employed 55 and older were classified as working part-time over the past four years because they cannot find full-time work or because of cutbacks in their customary hours.[9] The fraction of the older part-time employed who involuntarily work part-time tends to be higher among those under 55, among men, and among those with less education.[10]

A final labor market reserve is that of older workers with low weekly earnings, even when they are employed full-time. There are about 4.1 million full-time employed older persons (45-69) with weekly earnings below the four-person poverty line, equivalent to nearly 13% of all full-time employed older workers (1998-1999).[11] The incidence of low-wage problems among the older full-time employed tends to vary quite widely with the oldest and least well educated being the most likely to occupy low-wage jobs.

These four labor pools define a universe of 7.6 million older workers available to meet labor scarcities (Table 4).[12] This older worker labor reserve represents one in six of all older workers 45-69 and about 5% of the entire U.S. labor force. However, it is also a reserve that is particularly in need of employment and training services to prepare it for emerging skill needs.[13]

THE CASE OF OLDER WORKERS AND FULL EMPLOYMENT IN MASSACHUSETTS

The preceding description of the national labor reserve of older workers demonstrates both the growing importance of older persons to the economy and the magnitude of their employment difficulties, even in a prosperous economy. The national data, however, somewhat obscure the true importance of older workers to a full employment economy and do not fully portray the obstacles to utilizing older worker labor reserves. For example, the national unemployment rate during the 1990s never fell below 4% so that the labor supply constraints on economic growth were never so severe nationally as they were in some states. In addition, there are wide differences among states in their workforce demographics, with the mountain region having a relatively young workforce compared to that of the northeast and midwest.

The issues surrounding older workers in a full employment economy are, therefore, best illustrated by looking at a specific regional labor market with very low unemployment, labor scarcities, and a growing share of older workers in its economy. We have chosen Massachusetts as our example because it has been at the leading edge of the full employment economy in the United States. Its unemployment rate fell from a high of nearly 9% during the recession of the early 1990s to below 3% in 2000, making it the state with fourth lowest unemployment rate in the country at that time. Its population is aging at a far faster rate than the national average, making it a bellwether for at least eight other states in the northeast and midwest that will experience a rapidly aging workforce during this decade. Massachusetts also has a diversified economy with a strong high-technology sector, and a diversified workforce in terms of both education levels and extent of employment disadvantages.

The Labor Supply Gap and Bottlenecks to Growth in Massachusetts

Absent the current recession, official state employment projections show that further job growth of over 1.1% a year could be achieved if

TABLE 4. Estimated Reserves of Older Persons (45-69) (Average of March 1998-March 1999, in Millions)

Age Group	(A) Adjusted Civilian Labor Force	(B) Unemployed	(C) Employed Part-Time for Economic Reasons	(D) Labor Force Reserve	(E) Works Full-Time at Poverty Wages	(F) Total B to E	(G) Total as a % of Adjusted Labor Force
45-69	45.250	1.348	1.068	1.031	4.143	7.591	16.8
45-54	29.067	.840	.679	.495	2.573	4.588	15.8
55-69	16.183	.508	.389	.536	1.570	3.003	18.6

Source: March 1998 and March 1999 CPS surveys, tabulations by Center for Labor Market Studies, Northeastern University.

Massachusetts faced no labor supply constraints. However, even the most optimistic labor force projections show that only one-third to one-half of this job growth can be realized under reasonable assumptions about future population growth and labor supply behavior. If left uncorrected, this shortfall in labor supply could choke off growth either by creating bottlenecks of critical skills or by raising the costs of doing business in Massachusetts as employers compete for scarce labor. Massachusetts will need at least 217,000 more workers by 2006, or about 7% of its current workforce, if it is to achieve its full growth potential, and this supply gap could rise to as high as 268,000 if labor force participation rates do not increase over their 1995 levels (Doeringer, Sum, & Terkla, 2000).[14]

Even these pessimistic projections understate the labor supply constraints on growth because they ignore the decline in average hours worked and the doubling of the fraction of older males who are employed in part-time jobs since 1970. If the share of the older male population in full-time jobs in 1970 had not fallen over time, Massachusetts would have over 120,000 additional older males holding full-time jobs, almost 30% more than were actually employed full time in 1996-97.

Options for Closing the Labor Supply Gap

Massachusetts, as is the case nationally, has few choices for closing the projected gap in its labor supply. Its pool of younger adult workers (ages 25-39) is nearly fully employed (with unemployment rates as low as 1% or 2% for young adults with bachelor's degrees) and there will be an absolute decline in this group of workers over the next five years as the baby bust generation ages. Massachusetts ranks among the top 20 states in terms of the participation of all women in the labor force, leaving only a small margin for further growth in the female labor supply. Attracting more young workers to the state is likely to be quite difficult and could raise the costs of doing business in Massachusetts (Sum et al., 1998). Further reliance on foreign immigrants is a possibility, but Massachusetts already ranks second highest in the nation in its reliance on immigrants for its labor force growth (Sum et al., 1999), and annual immigration quotas for skilled workers have been considerably oversubscribed in the past.

Studies commissioned by the Massachusetts Blue Ribbon Commission on Older Workers (MBRCOW), however, show that there is a large and growing reserve of older workers. The number of older persons 45-69 years of age in the state's population began rising in the mid-1990s, after being stable for two decades, and this trend will accelerate over the current decade as the baby boom generation ages (Doeringer, Sum, & Terkla, 2000). Barring unforeseen events, all of the net growth in the Massachusetts labor supply through the year 2006 will come from persons 45 and older, and these older workers are expected to account for an all time high of at least two out of five workers by 2010.

Closing the labor supply gap in Massachusetts will require a substantial increase of six to seven percentage points in the labor force participation rates of the older population beyond those increases already projected. A much higher fraction of older persons in Massachusetts will have to remain at work than has been the case in recent years, more and better jobs will have to be found for those who are unemployed and underemployed, and inducements will be needed to encourage some of those currently outside the labor force to return to work.

A starting point for filling the supply gap are the 47,000 older persons who are currently unemployed. Adding in the 33,000 "hidden unemployed" (those who want jobs, but have not actually looked for work), the 34,000 part-time older workers who want full-time work, and the over 84,000 older workers who are in full-time, but marginal, employment (jobs that pay less than the poverty line wage of $300 per week) brings the older worker labor reserve to 190,000, or about 6% of the total workforce.

This labor pool, by itself, is large enough to meet a very substantial fraction of the Commonwealth's emerging labor-supply needs. The balance could be met by increasing the incentives for older workers to remain in, and return to, the labor market through higher skills and earnings.

Labor Market Mismatches

Numbers alone, however, are not enough to remedy labor supply constraints on growth. There is a substantial mismatch between the education levels and skills of many persons in this older worker labor reserve and the requirements of the fastest growing, higher-wage jobs in the Massachusetts economy that must also be addressed. Closing the labor supply gap will require a major investment in skills if older worker labor reserves are to reduce skill bottlenecks and aspire to the kinds of jobs that provide incentives for older workers to choose work over retirement.

The education mismatch is evident from employment projections for 2006 prepared by the Massachusetts Division of Employment and Training, which show that job growth will be concentrated among high-end industries that require high-skilled labor and, to a lesser extent, among those industries at the lower-skilled end of the labor market (Massachusetts DET, 1999). High-end growth industries include computer software and related services, biotechnology, selected financial services, medical offices, and private education services. These sectors will continue to have a high proportion of professional, managerial, and technical jobs that typically require at least a college education. Specific skill mismatches are likely to be in professional and technical occupations, such as systems engineers, software developers, biotech specialists, and allied health and various technical specialists (Massachusetts DET, 1999). Other professional occupations, such as teaching, will face major labor needs for replacing retirees, as well as meeting growth in demand. While low-end growth industries, such as eating and drinking establishments, personal services, retailing, and home health care, can more easily accommodate workers with less education, recent occupational projections suggest that almost half of all net new jobs in the Commonwealth will require a bachelor's degree or higher (Massachusetts DET, 1999).

Substantial education and training will be required to employ older workers in these jobs. While today's cohort of older workers in Massachusetts is better educated than its predecessors, older workers as a group are not as well educated as the young adults who have been the main source of labor supply to growth companies in Massachusetts during the 1990s. For example, only 30% of workers 55 to 65 have at least a bachelor's degree, well below the 40% for workers 25 to 34 (Doeringer, Sum, & Terkla, 2000). Among underutilized older workers, one quarter of the unemployed and almost one-third of the underemployed lack a high school diploma or its equivalent. In addition, many of the older workers who will be available to fill these jobs have skills and experience acquired in manufacturing occupations and other industries that are expected to be shedding labor. Such out-of-date skills are already a significant barrier to the employment of older workers (Wagner & Bonham, 1998), and skill mismatches are likely to become even more severe.

Labor Scarcities and Workplace Adjustment

Labor scarcities and skill mismatches of the magnitude projected for Massachusetts will also impose major adjustment costs on employers in terms of higher wages needed to recruit scarce workers, additional training expenses, and a substantial reorientation of human resources practices. Testimony received by the MBRCOW shows that Massachusetts's employers accurately monitor the tightness of their labor markets and are concerned with recruitment difficulties in a full employment economy, but few appreciate the full extent to which future demographic changes are likely to compound the costs of adjusting to labor scarcities.

For example, young adults are the traditional source of new hires for most growth industries in Massachusetts, with young adults in the 25-39 age range being preferred because they have both recent education and some work experience. There will be steep declines in the number of these more experienced young adults as the "baby bust" generation matures, which will force employers to turn to nontraditional sources of entry workers (Doeringer, Sum, & Terkla, 2000).[15]

Some relief will be provided by modest growth by 2006 in the number of young adults with little work experience (those 20-24 years old). However, this increase will not be large enough to offset the decline in young adults with prior work experience so that there will not be enough relatively well-educated workers in their twenties and thirties to fill entry-level job vacancies. While the highest-wage employers will be able to continue to hire experienced young adults into their entry jobs, the majority of employers in Massachusetts will have to substitute at least some older workers for traditional entry workers.

These employers will need to learn how to hire and train older workers for entry jobs, and to make corresponding adjustments in promotion ladders, career paths, and fringe benefit packages if they are to accommodate a nontraditional entry-level workforce. Hiring and selection practices will have to be adapted to a workforce that has more experience, but less up-to-date education. Training and promotion practices will need to be attuned to differences in how recent graduates and experienced workers learn new job skills. Wage and fringe benefit structures will need to accommodate differences in the compensation preferences of younger and older workers, and more flexible working hours will be needed for older workers who have different family or caregiver responsibilities than younger workers

These changes may not come easily. Managers often regard their existing older workers as excellent assets to the firm–more hardworking, reliable, and motivated than their younger counterparts (Sterns & McDaniel, 1994)–and they give older workers very high marks for their use of good judgement, quality control, attendance, and low turnover (AARP, 1995). However, they are also concerned that older workers are less willing to adapt to changing workforce practices and technologies. One study noted that older workers are viewed as somewhat fearful of new technologies and somewhat difficult to attract to the growing number of positions involving computer use (Belous, 1990), even though the use of computers by workers over 50 has doubled since the mid-1980s (Friedberg, 1999). Other studies have found that many employers believe older workers have difficulty learning new skills and are poor candidates for job training (Costello, 1997). A generally optimistic study (AARP, 1995) also found that the majority of managers believe that older workers are less flexible, innovative, and adaptable to workplace change than younger workers.

Unfortunately, these negative employer perceptions are reflected in workplace training practices. Older workers are in fact far less likely than their younger counterparts to be trained by their employers. In a nationwide survey of almost 1,500 establishments, 70% of all employees had received some formal training during the previous year, while less than 51% of workers 55 and over had received such training (Frazis, Gittleman, Horrigan, & Joyce, 1998), and little of the training received by these older workers was occupationally oriented.[16]

Adjustments to Labor Market Policy in Massachusetts

Massachusetts is as well or better equipped as any other state to address these potential mismatches. It offers a diverse array of employment and training programs that are typical of those available nationally.

The types of short-term occupational training programs that have been operated under the Job Training Partnership Act (JTPA) remain available under the new WIA. There is a strong base of adult basic education programs, which provide instruction in literacy and basic skills up to the high school level, and a community college system that offers both general education and advanced skills training. Subsidized part-time work experience opportunities are also available for low-income individuals 55 and older through the Senior Community Service Employment Program (SCSEP) and a few other modest state/federal programs for older workers. These programs, however, fall far short of the minimum needed to train older workers to fill the skill bottlenecks of a full employment economy.

The combined total of all federally supported short-term training programs, training for displaced workers, and subsidized community service jobs only provide resources sufficient to serve approximately 1 in 100 of the older persons in Massachusetts who can meet the relatively restrictive eligibility requirements for these programs. This shortfall in resources persisted during the boom economy of the late 1990s, when low unemployment and underemployment reduced the pool of eligible trainees (Doeringer, Sum, & Terkla, 2000). In practice, older workers do not even receive their full share of these limited resources because they are underrepresented in many programs, and when accepted into programs, they are more likely to receive counseling and placement services than more costly training.

This lack of resources is further compounded by the patchwork character of federal and state programs. Programs are funded under many different statutory authorizations and often have inconsistent eligibility requirements, making it difficult for participants to assemble a systematic sequence of counseling, education, training, and job placement services from among the different programs that are available. Inadequate standards for measuring program performance and inadequate funding for evaluating programs have also made quality control a problem. With the exception of JTPA and the new WIA programs, there has been no provision for systematic evaluation or follow-up activities to determine what works and what does not. Even the JTPA performance data covered only the first 90 days of post-training labor market experience and the post-program tracking of employment and earnings under WIA is limited 6 to 9 months, so that little is known about the long term consequences of training.

The limited information available from evaluations of JTPA programs shows that employment outcomes for older program participants in Massachusetts are relatively favorable, when compared with older workers nationally, at least in the short-term (see Table 5). For example, approximately 70% of all older persons terminating from Massachusetts JTPA Title IIA programs in Program Year 1996 were able to obtain employment, compared to 62% nationally. The employment rates for older Title III participants have also been higher in Massachusetts than nationally (72% vs. 68%). Likewise, wages received by older workers following training have consistently and substantially exceeded those nationally.

Unfortunately, the strong performance JTPA programs in Massachusetts, as compared to many other states, conceals the seriousness of the obstacles to upgrading the employment and earnings prospects of older workers. For example, only about three-fourths of all displaced workers 45 years of age and over who concluded their training in 1998 obtained employment. While the median wage replacement rate for these reemployed older workers was relatively high, one-third of those placed in jobs had wage losses of 20% or more and over one-fifth had wage losses of 30% or more. Data for New England during the mid-1990s show that these reemployment and wage replacement rates are substantially below the rates for younger dislocated workers under 45 and are lowest for older workers lacking high school diplomas.

MEETING THE POLICY CHALLENGES

The Massachusetts experience with a full employment economy clearly illustrates the extent to which labor scarcities and skill mismatches can limit economic growth. Older workers (age 45+), whose ranks are growing rapidly, provide the largest known labor reserve, both in Massachusetts and nationally, for avoiding these skill scarcities and labor supply deficits. Utilizing this reserve more effectively, however, means deferring retirement, bringing older persons back into the labor market, and increasing full-time employment. Too little funding, an emphasis on short-term programs, lack of coordination among programs, weak linkages to the private sector, and the limited flexibility in the human resources practices of large firms have left both government programs and employers ill-prepared to begin utilizing older worker labor reserves.

Despite this critique of employment and training policy, neither a return to federal governance nor radically different program designs are needed to address labor scarcities, skill mismatches, and low wages for older workers. Employment and training policy fared no better under federal leadership than it has under devolution to state and local govern-

TABLE 5. Selected Employment and Wage Outcomes for Older Persons (45-69) Terminating from JTPA Title IIA, Title III and Section 204 (d) Programs (Program Year 1996)

Programs	Employment Rate		Median Hourly Wage at Placement		Mean Hourly Wage at Followup	
	(A) U.S.	(B) Massachusetts	(A) U.S.	(B) Massachusetts	(A) U.S.	(B) Massachusetts
JTPA IIA	62.3	70.3	$7.00	$8.25	$7.73	$8.75
JTPA III	67.9	71.7	$9.37	$11.20	$11.47	$15.36
Section 204 (d)	62.5	69.7	$6.00	$8.00	$6.87	$8.75

Source: PY 1996 SPIR Information System, tabulations by the Center for Labor Market Studies.

ment, and the range of current programs is sufficiently large to provide a more than adequate set of building blocks from which an effective older worker labor market policy can be fashioned.

The biggest problems are that too few older workers are being trained to make a dent in our estimated 7% labor supply gap and that training programs are not substantial enough to make a difference in the skills and wages of older workers (Doeringer, Sum, & Terkla, 2000). For example, computer training has been a popular skill area among older trainees in Massachusetts JTPA programs. However, comments from our focus groups of older workers who have participated in these training programs stressed that training should be sufficient to build a range of skills, such as word processing, working with spreadsheets, graphic design, and manufacturing-related computer capacities, rather than on short-term computer literacy as is often the case. The overall conclusion from these groups is that training should be more comprehensive and directly transferable to jobs, not that new types of programmatic interventions are needed.[17]

Similarly, a much better understanding of the training needs of Massachusetts employers is required if they are to alter their current staffing patterns to include labor reserves of older workers. As the supply of experienced young adults dwindles, employers will have to find new ways to retain older employees, and many will have to turn to older workers to fill their entry jobs. Such staffing changes will require new approaches to recruitment, selection, training, and retirement policies that must be tailored to individual workplaces. These are issues that have not been considered by either the public training system in Massachusetts, or by employers themselves. Small employers (those with fewer than 50 employees) in particular are likely to face the most severe problems of adapting to older worker labor reserves because they employ more than their share of older workers and often lack the human resources development capacity of large, private-sector companies.

Massachusetts has taken a useful step to correct some of the deficiencies in workplace training by enacting a "Workforce Training Fund," financed by unemployment insurance monies, to help employers train incumbent workers. However, this program is only modestly funded and, like many other training programs, its effectiveness has not been evaluated.

Identifying emerging skill scarcities, assessing what training is needed to bridge the skill and education mismatches between older workers and the new jobs being generated by employers, and working closely with employers and unions to close the labor supply gap require a network of employment centers that can work on both the supply and the demand sides of the labor market. The WIA model of one-stop career centers linked together through statewide coordination and evaluation mechanisms is potentially suited to play this role, but its functions, including information gathering on applicants, job orders, and successful job matching, will have to be improved considerably.

What is critical to making this model work, however, is the political commitment to fund and implement a coherent workforce development system of sufficient size and accountability to improve substantially the skills, wages, and work incentives of older workers. By focusing on job quality and higher wage incentives, employment and training policy can address both the growth and business competitiveness problems of labor scarcities and the social problems of poverty and income inadequacy. The new WIA provides a fresh opportunity to move in this direction, and this same model needs to be extended to the entire workforce development system.

There is a broad consensus among employers, workers, policy analysts, and employment and training professionals around a set of principles for building an active and effective labor market policy at the state and local levels that can serve the skill needs of both workers and employers in a full employment economy (Doeringer, Sum, & Terkla, 2000). These include (1) focusing all elements of workforce development on achieving high quality job placements and long-term upgrading of the workforce in order to raise earnings and strengthen work incentives; (2) harmonizing program eligibility and training content among the different programs so that older workers can more easily accumulate higher levels of education and skill during their extended work careers; (3) targeting program resources on alleviating skill scarcities and mismatches; (4) strengthening workforce development through public-private partnerships with employers and unions; (5) establishing an evaluation process that provides both long-term tracking of program terminees' labor market experiences and continuous improvement of the performance of workforce development programs; and (6) providing the additional financial resources needed to close the labor supply gap under full employment conditions.

NOTES

1. Separate funding streams remain under Title One for youth, adults (22 and older), and dislocated workers.

2. The major exceptions are the Job Corps and the national Urban Service Corps (Schochet et al., 2000).

3. Our upper age cutoff of 69 is used since labor force participation rates for workers in their early 70s are very low and few express a desire for jobs. Only 14% of all persons 70-74 were active in the labor force of the nation in 2001, and only slightly more than 1% of those out-of-the labor force expressed a desire for an immediate job.

4. These findings are based on tabulations performed by the Center for Labor Market Studies on the January 1998-December 1999 CPS surveys. The unemployment rates of 45-64 year olds were below 3% at the end of the 1990s, the lowest of all age groups. Over the 1998-99 period, the average monthly unemployment rate for 45-54 year olds ranged from a high of 6.2% for those older workers with only a primary education to a low of 1.7% for those who had obtained a bachelor's or higher degree. Similar, though somewhat less extreme, unemployment differentials prevailed for workers in the 55-64 and 65 and older subgroups.

5. For earlier reviews of the labor market problems of older workers in the United States and Massachusetts, see Sum and Fogg, 1991; Sum and Fogg, 1998.

6. These "hidden unemployed" who are not working and not looking for work, but want a job, should not be confused with the BLS concept of a "discouraged worker" who must also meet certain job search and workforce availability tests. Such discouraged workers are only a small subset of the hidden unemployed or labor force reserve, typically under 10% in recent years.

7. The share of the economically inactive population desiring immediate employment tends to decline uniformly with age. In 1998, 16% of the 16-24 year old members of the economically inactive population were members of the labor force reserve versus 11% of those 25-54 and only 2% of those 55 and older.

8. These estimates are based on the 1998 and 1999 CPS surveys. The tendency for employed 65-69 year olds to work part-time was undoubtedly influenced by the Social Security earnings penalty test, which reduced Social Security benefits by one-third for all earnings above a specific threshold. The U.S. Congress has recently eliminated this earnings penalty for those 65-69.

9. BLS classifies an individual as part-time for economic reasons only if he or she cites a desire for full-time work and reports that he or she was available for full-time

work during the reference week of the survey. In Table 4, we report all persons working part-time for economic reasons regardless of their availability for full-time work. Men were somewhat more likely than women to be working part-time for economic reasons in each year.

10. On average, over the 1998-99 period, approximately 13% of 45-54-year-old part-time workers were employed part-time for economic reasons versus only 9% of those 55-69. These estimates are based solely on reasons cited by the older workers for working part-time and do not take into account their current availability for full-time work.

11. In 1998, the average poverty threshold for a four-person family in the United States was slightly above $16,600; thus, to avoid being poor, a full-time, year-round employed family head would have needed gross weekly earnings of approximately $320. These estimates are somewhat conservative due to the fact that the CPS survey only collects weekly earnings data from wage and salary workers. Some members of the self-employed also will experience low wage problems during the year but they cannot be identified with the CPS weekly earnings data.

12. The official labor force statistics exclude the members of the labor force reserve. Our adjusted labor force includes the employed, unemployed, and the members of the labor force reserve.

13. The findings of the March 1998 and March 1999 national CPS household surveys were combined to estimate the number of 45-69 year olds experiencing one of these four mutually exclusive types of labor market problems.

14. 217,000 reflects the difference between the projected growth in state employment (12%) and the most optimistic projected growth (5.9%) in the resident labor force, which leaves a 6.1 percentage point (of approximately a 3.2 million labor force) gap. Foreign immigrants have accounted for all net labor force growth in the state between 1990 and 2000.

15. The cohort of workers 25-39 years old will shrink by more than 200,000 between 1995 and the year 2005.

16. The survey also suggests that training rates are about 50% higher for college graduates than for employees with a high school education or less and that a disproportionate share of employer training goes to managerial and professional occupations.

17. Recent findings from Pennsylvania on the post-program experiences of older dislocated workers enrolled in community college programs show very little return from such training unless it is very occupational specific and job-oriented (LaLonde et al., 2001).

AUTHOR NOTES

Peter Doeringer is Professor of Economics at Boston University and has taught at Harvard University, the London School of Economics, and the University of Paris. His research interests include labor markets, collective bargaining, industry economics, and regional economic development. He serves regularly as a consultant and adviser to government agencies and international organizations, most recently as Director of Research for the Commonwealth of Massachusetts Blue Ribbon Commission on Older Workers. Professor Doeringer is also a practicing labor arbitrator.

Dr. Doeringer can be contacted at the Department of Economics, Boston University, 270 Bay State Road, Boston, MA 02125 (E-mail: doeringe@bu.edu).

Andrew Sum is Professor of Economics at Northeastern University and Director of the Center for Labor Market Studies in Boston. He has been involved with employment and training policymaking, planning, and evaluation at the local, state, and national levels for nearly three decades. He has numerous publications on the economies of New England and Massachusetts and in the areas of youth labor market problems, employment and training policies, older workers, and literacy issues. He has recently served on the research staff for the Commonwealth's Blue Ribbon Commission on Older Workers.

Professor Sum can be contacted at the Department of Economics, Northeastern University, 301 Lake Hall, Boston, MA 02115-5000 (E-mail: a.sum@neu.edu).

David Terkla is Professor of Economics at the University of Massachusetts Boston and a senior fellow in the Gerontology Institute. His research interests include environmental economics, regional economic development, and industry economics and management practices. He is active in advising government agencies on regional economic development issues and fishery management policy and has recently served on the research staff for the Commonwealth's Blue Ribbon Commission on Older Workers.

Professor Terkla can be contacted at the Department of Economics, University of Massachusetts Boston, 100 Morrissey Blvd., Boston, MA 02215-3393 (E-mail: david.terkla@umb.edu).

This article draws, in part, on materials from the authors' previous work on *Older Workers: An Essential Resource for Massachusetts* (2000) (the final report of the Commonwealth of Massachusetts Blue Ribbon Commission on Older Workers, for which the authors served as research staff) and "Older Workers and Active Labour Market Policy in a Full Employment Economy," in Hedva Sarfati and Giuliano Bonoli (Eds.) *Labour Market and Social Protection Reforms in International Perspective: Parallel or Converging Tracks?* (Aldershot, UK: Ashgate Publishing, 2002). The authors want to acknowledge the assistance of Alison Gottlieb of the University of Massachusetts Boston and Neeta Fogg, Neal Fogg, Sheila Palma, Steve Rubb, and Paul Suozzo of Northeastern University. This version of the study benefited from the comments of an anonymous reviewer.

REFERENCES

AARP (1995). *Valuing Older Workers: A Study of Costs and Productivity.* Washington, DC: AARP.

Belous, R. S. (1990). Flexible employment: The employer's point of view. In Peter B. Doeringer (Ed.), *Bridges To Retirement: Older Workers in a Changing Labor Market.* Ithaca, NY: Cornell University Press.

Costello, C. (1997). *Training Older Workers for the Future.* Cambridge, MA: Radcliff Public Policy Institute, Radcliff College

Doeringer, P. B. et al. (1991). *Turbulence in the American Work Place.* New York, NY: Oxford University Press.

Doeringer, P. B., Sum, A., & Terkla, D. (2000). *Older Workers: An Essential Resource for Massachusetts.* Boston: The Massachusetts Blue Ribbon Commission on Older Workers.

Frazis, H., Gittleman, M., Horrigan, M., & Joyce, M. (1998). Results from the 1995 survey of employer-provided training. *Monthly Labor Review*, June, pp. 3-13.

Friedberg, L. K. (1999). The Impact of Technological Change on Older Workers. NBER Working Paper, University of San Diego and NBER, February.

Fullerton, H. Jr. (1999). Labor force projections to 2008. *Monthly Labor Review*, November.

LaLonde, R., Jacobson, L., & Sullivan, D. G. (2001). The Returns to Community College Schooling for Displaced Workers. Westat Inc. and NBER, January.

Mangum, G., Mangum, S., & Sum, A. (1998). *A Fourth Chance for Second Chance Programs: Lessons from the Old for the New*. Sar Levitan Center for Social Policy Studies, Johns Hopkins University, Baltimore.

Massachusetts Division of Employment and Training (DET) (1999). The Massachusetts Job Outlook Through 2006. Boston.

Mucciaroni, G. (1990). *The Political Failure of Employment Policy, 1945-1982*. Pittsburgh, PA: The University of Pittsburgh Press.

National Council on Aging (2000). *Myths and Realities of Aging: Comparison of 1974 Survey to 2000 Survey Results*.

Orr, L. L., Bloom, H. S. et al. (1996). *Does Training for the Disadvantaged Work? Evidence from the National JTPA Study*. Washington, DC: The Urban Institute Press.

Schochet, P. et al. (2000). *National Job Corps Study: The Short-Term Impacts of Job Corps on Participants' Employment and Related Outcomes*. Princeton, NJ: Mathematica Policy Research, Inc., February.

Sterns, H. L., & McDaniel, M. A. (1994). Job performance and the older worker. In S.E. Rix (Ed.), *Older Workers: How Do They Measure Up? An Overview of Age Differences in Employee Costs and Performance*. Washington, DC: AARP.

Sum, A. et al. (1999). *The Changing Workforce: Immigrants and the New Economy in Massachusetts*. Boston: The Massachusetts Institute for a New Commonwealth.

Sum, A., Bahuguna, A., Fogg, N., Fogg, W., Harrington, P., Palma, S., & Suozzo, W. (1998). *The Road Ahead: Emerging Threats to Workers, Families, and the Massachusetts Economy*. Boston: Teresa and H. John Heinz Foundation and MassINC.

Sum, A., & Fogg, W. N. (1998). *The Labor Market Problems of Older Workers in the Late 1990s in Massachusetts and the U.S.* Boston: Research Paper prepared for the Massachusetts Blue Ribbon Commission on Older Workers.

Sum, A., & Fogg, W. N. (1991). Labor market turbulence and the older Worker. In P.B. Doeringer (Ed.), *Turbulence in the American Workplace*. New York, NY: Oxford University Press.

U. S. Census Bureau (2000). *Population Projections to 2050*. Website.

U. S. Department of Labor, Bureau of Labor Statistics (2000). *Worker Displacement During the Late 1990s*. Washington, DC, August.

Wagner, D. L., & Bonham, G. S. (1998). "Factors Influencing the Use of Older Workers: A Survey of U.S. Employers." Paper delivered at Gerontological Society of America, Annual Scientific Conference, Philadelphia, PA, November.

Volunteerism and Social Capital in Policy Implementation: Evidence from the Long-Term Care Ombudsman Program

Andrew B. Whitford, PhD

University of Kansas

Jeff Yates, JD, PhD

University of Georgia

SUMMARY. We assess the link between a program's volunteer support and state social capital in the case of the joint implementation of the federal Long-Term Care (LTC) Ombudsman Program by state and federal authorities. This program, which is designed to prevent elder abuse and ensure quality care in long-term facilities, is implemented at the state and local levels and relies heavily on volunteer staff. First, we find that volunteerism is vital to the efficacy of the program's monitoring and investigative functions. Second, we find that volunteerism in this program is tied to broader level conditions of a state's social capital. Last, we discuss the implications of our findings for volunteer-based programs devolved to the states. *[Article copies available for a fee from The Haworth Document Delivery Service: 1-800-HAWORTH. E-mail address: <getinfo@haworthpressinc.com> Website: <http://www.HaworthPress.com> © 2002 by The Haworth Press, Inc. All rights reserved.]*

[Haworth co-indexing entry note]: "Volunteerism and Social Capital in Policy Implementation: Evidence from the Long-Term Care Ombudsman Program." Whitford, Andrew B., and Jeff Yates. Co-published simultaneously in *Journal of Aging & Social Policy* (The Haworth Press, Inc.) Vol. 14, No. 3/4, 2002, pp. 61-73; and: *Devolution and Aging Policy* (ed: Francis G. Caro, and Robert Morris) The Haworth Press, Inc., 2002, pp. 61-73. Single or multiple copies of this article are available for a fee from The Haworth Document Delivery Service [1-800-HAWORTH, 9:00 a.m. - 5:00 p.m. (EST). E-mail address: getinfo@haworthpressinc.com].

10.1300/J031v14n03_04

KEYWORDS. Social capital, volunteerism, policy implementation, long-term care, federalism

INTRODUCTION

The Long-Term Care Ombudsman Program is a federal project falling under the Older Americans Act (OAA), whereby staff and volunteer ombudsmen advocate on the behalf of older residents of long-term care (LTC) facilities. The programs are located in every state and many regional or local areas, and assist residents and their families in obtaining quality care in nursing homes, assisted living, and other types of LTC facilities. Ombudsmen identify, investigate, and work to help resolve individual and systematic complaints by the residents of LTC facilities (Huber et al., 2001, 61). The value of this program lies in staff advocacy and the representation of residents' interests, since residents may be unable to press claims due to minimal resources or diminished capacity. This federal program is overseen by the Administration on Aging (AoA) in the U.S. Department of Health and Human Services and is implemented by state, local, and other (private or non-profit) entities. All of these organizations rely heavily on volunteer workers: in 1998, almost 90% of all ombudsmen were volunteers.

Our interest centers on unequal participation of volunteers in the ombudsman program across the states. Because volunteers identify code violations and advocate on the behalf of LTC residents, this federal program's national benefits depend explicitly on the individual states' commitment to and public participation in the program. As an example, in 1998, North Carolina fielded 1,232 volunteers, while Georgia fielded just 13.

First, we address the integral role that volunteers play in this jointly-implemented program. Second, we evaluate the proposition that the condition of social capital in states fundamentally constrains volunteerism in this program. Social capital can be thought of as a type of glue that holds communities together. At its core, a community's state of social capital is dictated by how networks of individuals in a community create conditions where people are inclined to do things for one other (Putnam, 2000). In a very real sense, social capital sets the bounds–or determines the likelihood–for "norms of reciprocity." It works in combination with information flows in networks, collective action, and broader identities and social solidarity among individuals. We argue that LTC volunteerism may be constrained, to a degree, by the state of civil society and social capital formation.

Our study focuses on the unequal distribution of volunteer personnel across the states. We examine the differences among states in volunteer ombudsman presence and argue that these disparities may be attributable to the broader macro-contextual characteristics of the states' citizens. This link between volunteerism and social capital means that the program's viability turns, at least in part, on state-level social factors outside the control of program designers. This assessment aids our understanding of how federal agencies implement programs through states and volunteers, how the quality of long-term care depends on this joint implementation, and what an aging population and federal devolution will mean for the future of quality long-term care in the United States.

THE OMBUDSMAN PROGRAM
AND THE ROLE OF VOLUNTEERS

The Long-Term Care Ombudsman Program began in the early 1970s as a set of demonstration programs in response to widespread concerns over the inadequate and sometimes abusive treatment of residents of nursing homes (Huber et al., 2000; Netting et al., 1995). By 1978 the Older Americans Act amendments mandated that all states operate a statewide ombudsman program, either directly or by contract (Netting et al., 1995). These programs are primarily funded by the federal government, with additional funds coming from state and local sources. The various state ombudsman programs are primarily implemented by a variety of designated Local Ombudsman Entities (LOEs), including regional offices of the state ombudsman programs, area agencies on aging, and free standing ombudsman programs, among others. These LOEs recruit and train volunteers, and largely implement this program.

Ombudsman responsibilities under the act include the following:

- identify, investigate, and resolve complaints made by or on behalf of residents;
- provide information to residents about long-term care services;
- represent the interests of residents before governmental agencies and seek administrative, legal, and other remedies to protect residents;
- analyze, comment on, and recommend changes in laws and regulations pertaining to the health, safety, welfare, and rights of residents;

- educate and inform consumers and the general public regarding issues and concerns related to long-term care, and facilitate public comment on laws, regulations, policies, and actions;
- promote the development of citizen organizations to participate in the program; and
- provide technical support for the development of resident and family councils to protect the well-being and rights of residents (Long-Term Care Ombudsman Report–FY 1998, Administration on Aging–Department of Health and Human Services).

The Act allows the states substantial discretion to structure their programs according to their own preferences and philosophies. State and substate programs may expand the scope and responsibility of volunteer efforts (such as working side-by-side with paid staff) or alternatively constrain volunteer roles to lesser types of responsibilities (see Huber et al., 2000; Netting et al., 1992; Netting et al., 1995). For instance, some ombudsman programs operate in a non-contest-oriented manner with volunteers playing rather neutral roles as mediators and resource brokers (e.g., New York) while other programs employ a tougher patient rights model that involves volunteers taking on contest-oriented roles as consumer advocates and watchdogs (e.g., Oregon) (Nelson, 1995). The ombudsmen are essentially external agents of quality assurance in LTC and, as such, provide an important community presence in LTC facilities (Cherry, 1993). Although ombudsman programs are implemented by both paid staff and volunteers, the vast majority of ombudsman program personnel are volunteers. The role, impact, and value of volunteers in state ombudsman programs have been frequent topics of professional discussion and study (see Huber et al., 1993).

The substantial variance in the role of volunteers in ombudsman programs among states (and within states)[1] has traditionally made assessments of the impact of volunteers on the quality of LTC care a challenging research endeavor. However, a general understanding of the role and impact of volunteers has emerged. Studies concerning volunteers in the ombudsman program have examined, among other things, the impact of volunteer presences on LTC quality of care (Nelson, 1995), the relationship between the extent of ombudsman volunteerism and complaint frequency (Nelson et al., 1995), and the impact of volunteer/paid staff mix on complaint reports and complaint resolutions (Huber et al., 1993). While the results of these studies are somewhat mixed, in part due to different study venues, we can reasonably link increased volunteerism to higher levels of reported and investigated complaints.

Certainly, increased monitoring activity does not dictate the quality of care for LTC residents and only represents one way of assessing program effectiveness. The debate over the determinants of LTC program effectiveness and quality of care outcomes are beyond the scope of this article. Here, we address only the important role of volunteers in the program. Generally, LTC professionals and academics agree that volunteerism is important to the vitality of the ombudsman program and quality care in LTC facilities.

VOLUNTEERISM AND SOCIAL CAPITAL

In recent years, social scientists have oriented on the value of "social capital" in communities. Perhaps more than any other concept recently in social science, social capital has caught the public imagination–both in terms of media attention and political action.[2] But in a real sense, social capital is connected to the underlying mechanisms and processes that determine the vitality of democracy, its institutions, and public organizations; this claim is as old as Tocqueville's *Democracy in America* analyses (Tocqueville, 1945). There are three common concerns in the literature on social capital: to explore the determinants of social capital; to document its decline in modern America; and to offer solutions (e.g., Putnam, 2000; Verba, Schlozman, & Brady, 1995). In large part, its determinants are marked by their coincidence with its decline. Social changes like the rise of commuting time coincide with decreases in club attendance, family dinners, and having friends over. Putnam tags this new state of affairs as "bowling alone."[3] Initiatives like Harvard's Saguaro Seminar on Civic Engagement have as a goal mitigating these societal shifts.

The LTC Ombudsman Program is fundamentally *volunteer-dependent*. Indeed, without volunteerism, surveillance and advocacy are simply goals because this program is resource poor. To our knowledge, no federal enforcement program makes as extensive use of volunteers as this one does. Volunteer labor provides a direct substitute for the federal commitment of resources; while there are paid staff and states surely supplement federal outlays, the personnel are primarily volunteers. The central problem, of course, is that rates of volunteerism vary across states. The precept of the social capital enterprise is that volunteerism depends on social capital, and that different areas have different levels of capital. While there may have been a general decline in capital over time, a central result of Putnam's project is to document variations in the state of social capital across areas of the United States.

We combine two primary data sources in our analysis. Our data on LTC Ombudsman volunteerism come from the U.S. Department of Health and Human Services Administration on Aging (AoA). The AoA provides yearly data on the states' implementation of the Ombudsman program, including detailed information on volunteer involvement and activities. We use data from four years–Fiscal Years 1996 to 1999–that come from the AoA's Annual Reports and Reporting System Data Tables.[4] We examine the activities and involvement of volunteers across the 50 states for the four years. Because our interest is in the overall implementation of this joint federal-state-volunteer program, we move beyond the traditional use of single or limited numbers of states, or reliance on specific years of data. We recognize that our point about state-level variation in implementation and volunteer involvement is cross-sectional, but we use multiple year-level observations for each state to provide a more complete picture of the underlying mechanisms.

Our second data source is a collection of state-level measurements of social capital gathered by Putnam.[5] Putnam provides these measurements to allow for multiple mechanisms and views of social capital across the 50 states. Our measures include a range of limited indicators of social capital (ranging from time spent volunteering to the presidential turnout) and a broad "social capital index" for more general statements about the connection between social capital and volunteerism. The advantage here is that we tap into both broad notions of social capital in the 50 states and into dimensions of social capital construction that may be useful for program designers when relying on volunteerism for the implementation of similar programs.

Our primary measure of volunteerism is the percentage of people involved in a state's LTC Ombudsman program who are volunteers. By volunteers, we include both Certified Volunteer Ombudsmen (CVOs) and "Other Volunteers" reported by the states. Volunteers are compared to the total number of involved people, which includes paid program staff (PPS). Figure 1 shows that for 1999, this volunteer percentage varies widely across the states. For the entire time period, the average is 71.7% and the standard deviation is 32.0. The maximum is 99.90%; the minimum is 0.0%. Additionally, it is notable that the variance for the number of volunteers in a state is much higher than the variance for the number of paid staff per state.[6] One implication of this is that if the states want to expand their enforcement efforts, a practical option is to expand their volunteer base.

While the mass of the distribution is at the upper end of the measure's range, there remains clear variation in volunteerism across the states. This measure–the mixture of volunteers and program staff–provides an indication of the degree to which the program is aided, or complemented, by community presence (i.e., volunteers) (see Huber et al., 1993).

As others have argued (Nelson, 1995; Nelson et al., 1995; Huber et al., 1993; Cherry, 1991), the degree of volunteer presence (mixture of volunteers) in a LTC facility is tied to higher rates of problem identification and investigations. Implicitly, this monitoring and investigation activity leads to higher quality LTC care in the long run (Huber et al., 1993). Specifically, Cherry suggests that along with the more tangible aspects of monitoring and investigation, volunteer presence may act as a professionalizing stimulant for paid staff by enhancing staff pride in their work, and that staff may also feel more accountable due to the watchdog function of volunteers (Cherry, 1991, 302).

FIGURE 1. The Extent of States' LTC Volunteer Presence (Volunteers as a Percentage of all LTC Staff–1999 Data)

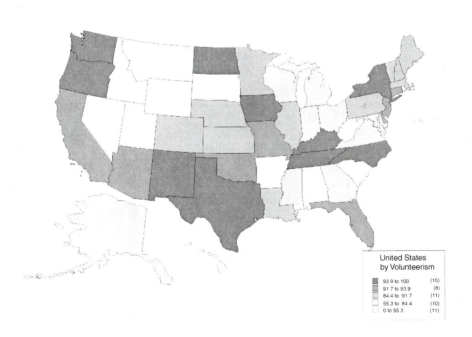

United States
by Volunteerism

	93.9 to 100	(10)
	91.7 to 93.9	(8)
	84.4 to 91.7	(11)
	55.3 to 84.4	(10)
	0 to 55.3	(11)

Our analyses corroborate these studies by showing a direct relationship between our measure of volunteer presence (composition) and monitoring productivity, measured by case-opening and complaint-handling. As Table 1 shows, the number of cases opened is higher when the percentage of volunteers is higher; the number of complaints recorded is also higher.[7] This is important for two reasons. First, volunteerism has a measurable impact on the productivity of these programs, in terms of their monitoring and investigative attributes. Second, our data are reasonable, in that they comport with the standard findings in the LTC gerontology literature detailed above.

On the whole, the LTC Ombudsman program depends on volunteerism across the states for its viability. Unlike many other programs, this joint implementation by the states and the federal government–through volunteers–is shaped by the level of social capital across the states. Table 2 shows that the mix of volunteers–shown to be a key determinant of the program's monitoring effectiveness–is conditioned on the level of social capital in a state.[8] Our first piece of evidence is the relationship between the volunteer percentage and Putnam's broad social capital index (Row 1). The importance of this result is that volunteerism is broadly connected to social capital *measured at its most aggregated level*. This means that LTC monitoring effectiveness is fundamentally constrained by volunteerism, and volunteerism is a function of the state of reciprocity and social networks in local areas. For program design, the uniform implementation of this program is highly unlikely, as long as different local social networks vary in their strength, broadness, and depth of interactions.

Table 2 also reveals how different aspects of social capital formation affect the mix of volunteer involvement in the LTC Ombudsman program across the states. The percentage of volunteers is associated with factors including statewide survey responses on questions about time spent entertaining and volunteering, service in local clubs and committees, attendance at town meetings, and "whether most people can be trusted." Volunteerism also correlates with the mean presidential turnout in a state.[9] Most notably, the strongest correlations are for the measures tapping into time spent volunteering and entertaining; these measures are most directly related to both volunteerism in the generic sense, and the volunteerism that underpins the Ombudsman program. The importance of these results is that these measures–unlike the social capital index–are directly observable by program designers, who can relate their design decisions to variations in the state of specific aspects in local areas. Specifically, the likelihood of volunteerism (in terms of

TABLE 1. Prais-Winsten Regression Estimates of the Effect of Volunteer Presence (Volunteers as a Percentage of All LTC Staff) on Two Measures of Monitoring Productivity

Variables	Cases Opened Coefficient Estimate	Complaints Handled Coefficient Estimate
Volunteer Presence	6.288** (2.413)	6.864** (2.606)
Number of Facilities in State	1.373** (0.251)	1.744** (0.355)
Constant	632.954* (270.149)	1304.829** (450.011)
R^2	0.296	0.302
N	200	200
ρ	0.810	0.809

(Standard Errors in Parentheses)

* indicates significance at better than 0.05 (one-tailed test).
** indicates significance at better than 0.01 (one-tailed test).

Note: analysis performed using STATA 7.0.

survey evidence of time spent volunteering) is an indicator of the likely mix of volunteers in a state, and, thus, the long-term effectiveness of the program.[10] Working backwards, social capital bounds volunteerism and volunteerism constrains monitoring functions in the LTC Ombudsman program.

CONCLUSIONS

What do these relationships mean for long-term care in the United States? We believe there are three broad implications. First, states with low social capital may suffer from inadequate program staffing, unless they are willing to substitute for volunteerism with greater resources for LTC programs. Of course, it may be the case that even now such a substitution occurs. Even so, past studies and our data show that volunteerism is a key determinant of program monitoring success. And, of course, such substitution turns on the ability and willingness of states to subsidize the program. Hence, the devolution of implementation to the states entails the federal program releasing some degree of control and uniformity.

TABLE 2. Robust Correlations for Volunteer Presence (Volunteers as a Percentage of All LTC Staff) and Eight Measures of Social Capital

Social Capital Measures	Volunteer Presence	
	Correlation	Bias-Corrected Numerical Confidence Interval
Putnam's Social Capital Index	0.2056**	[0.0338,0.3476]
Times Entertained at Home	0.3400***	[0.1814,0.4672]
Times Volunteered Last Year	0.2979***	[0.1657,0.4191]
Served on Committee for Local Organization	0.1982**	[0.0382,0.3157]
Served as Officer of Club or Organization	0.2024**	[0.0581,0.3300]
Attended a Meeting in Town or School Affairs	0.2191**	[0.0929,0.3274]
Trust in People	0.1980*	[0.0004,0.3504]
Presidential Turnout	0.2382***	[0.0774,0.3672]

N = 200

* indicates significance at better than 0.05 (two-tailed test).
** indicates significance at better than 0.01 (two-tailed test).
*** indicates significance at better than 0.001 (two-tailed test).

Second, future growth in the elderly population over time will likely mean an escalating need for this program. Because of the links between volunteerism and effectiveness, and between social capital and volunteerism, program effectiveness is bounded, to some degree, by a mechanism that is largely uncontrollable by the program designers. Increases in need must be matched by increases in volunteerism; increased volunteerism would require increases in social capital. This conditional nature of a devolved LTC program (through volunteerism) may not suffice.

Third, this unequal distribution of volunteerism across states may be at least partially subsumed by a larger trend: the general decline in social capital. While our data do not have the time span to investigate this point, social science's primary concern about social capital is its general decline–not its linkage to any one social program. While the LTC Ombudsman program is advantaged in some local areas by their relative wealth of social capital, all areas are losing social capital at alarming rates. The expected growth of the LTC population and the continued reliance of this program on volunteers indicate that disadvantaged areas will likely remain disadvantaged, and that advantaged areas will face stiff opposition to improvements.

Putnam's call for bolstering social capital (Putman, 2000, 402-14) has some relevance for the vitality of the LTC Ombudsman program. He argues that improving social capital in this country depends on both individual level resourcefulness and systematic institutional initiatives; his litany of suggestions includes advances in youth civic education and opportunities, the workplace environment, and government reform. In sum, improving social capital will require the reconsideration and revision of many of the practices and policies of modern America. If these proposals bolstered civic engagement generally, we might see a correlated increase in volunteer assistance in the LTC Ombudsman program. One micro-level initiative could be to increase volunteer recruiting efforts–but, of course, this would also require expanded resource outlays and might have only marginal effects. Yet, these broader social trends largely are beyond the control of LTC administrators. But recognizing social capital's role in volunteerism can help administrators in their search for other, more proximate answers to the needs of this fundamental program for the aged.

NOTES

1. While we explicitly acknowledge the intrastate variance in the role of volunteers in LTC programs, an in-depth analysis of this issue is beyond the scope of this study, which focuses on the interstate differences in volunteer roles and participation.

2. For instance, see the Civic Practices Network at http://www.cpn.org.

3. Ostensibly, the title and tag line of Putnam's book, *Bowling Alone*, is derived at least in part from a story that he relates that goes to the core of his theory and argument. In short, he tells the story of two men whose only connection is being in the same bowling league, but that this simple connection leads one of the men to donate his kidney to the other. Putnam notes, "[t]his moving story speaks for itself, but the photograph that accompanied this report in the *Ann Arbor News* reveals that in addition to their differences in profession and generation, Boschma is white and Lambert is African American. That they bowled together made all the difference. In small ways like this–and in larger ways too–we Americans need to reconnect with one another. That is the simple argument of this book" (2000, 28).

4. These reports are publicly available at http://www.aoa.gov/ltcombudsman/default.htm.

5. Putnam's data are available at http://www.bowlingalone.com.

6. For 1999, the mean number of volunteers per state was 284.70 with a standard deviation of 615.20; the mean number of paid staff per state for that year was 19.22 with a standard deviation of 20.03.

7. We control for the size of the nursing home population by including the number of facilities in the state. Our data are constructed as a wide panel, so we estimate the con-

ditional relationship of volunteer presence on our two monitoring productivity measures by Prais-Winsten regression (with panel-corrected standard errors, see Beck & Katz, 1995). In this case, we account for the time-series nature of the dependent variable by estimating an autocorrelation parameter (p); it is large in each case. These inferences are also based on Huber-White robust standard errors.

8. We recognize that the limited number of state-years involved in our samples may result in a type of fragility. To bolster these results, we bootstrapped these statistics to produce numerical confidence intervals (CIs) (reproduced in the right-hand column of Table 1). Following convention, we report bias-corrected CIs from 1000 replications of the calculation of each statistic (each replication is calculated based on 200 observations resampled with replacement). See Mooney and Duval (1993) for full details on resampling techniques.

9. Putnam (2000) discusses these factors at length (Table 4 and pp. 290-291).

10. To confirm the robustness of the tie between social capital and volunteerism, we ran an auxiliary model using an alternative measure of volunteerism–the total number of volunteers per capita in the state. We found that this measure is positively correlated with these same measures of social capital (those in Table 2). These correlations are significant at the 0.10 level of significance (two-tailed test) or better.

AUTHOR NOTES

Andrew B. Whitford is Assistant Professor of Political Science at the University of Kansas. His recent research centers on bureaucratic politics and policy implementation in the areas of regulation and environmental, health, and energy policy.

Dr. Whitford can be contacted at the Department of Political Science, University of Kansas, 504 Blake Hall, 1541 Lilac Lane, Lawrence, KS 66044 (E-mail: whitford@ku.edu).

Jeff Yates is an attorney and Assistant Professor in the Political Science Department at the University of Georgia. He is the author of *Popular Justice* (Albany: SUNY Press) and has also published articles on judicial politics, criminal justice, and aging policy.

Dr. Yates can be contacted at the Department of Political Science, University of Georgia, Athens, GA 30602 (E-mail: jyates@arches.uga.edu).

REFERENCES

Beck, N., & Katz, J. N. (1995). What to do (and not to do) with time-series cross-section data. *American Political Science Review, 89,* 634-647.

Cherry, R. L. (1991). Agents of nursing home quality of care: Ombudsmen and staff ratios revisited. *The Gerontologist, 31,* 302-308.

Cherry, R. L. (1993). Community presence and nursing home quality of care: The ombudsman as a complementary role. *Journal of Health and Social Behavior, 34,* 336-45.

Huber, R., Borders, K., Netting, F. E., & Kautz, J. R. (2000). Interpreting the meaning of ombudsman data across states: The critical analyst-practitioner link. *Journal of Applied Gerontology, 19,* 3-22.

Huber, R., Borders, K., Netting, F. E., & Nelson, H. W. (2001). Data from long-term care ombudsman programs in six states: The implications of collecting resident demographics. *The Gerontologist, 41*, 61-8.

Huber, R., Netting, F. E., & Patton, R. N. (1993). In search of the impact of staff mix on long-term care ombudsman programs. *Nonprofit and Public Sector Quarterly, 22*, 69-91.

Mooney, C. Z., & Duval, R. D. (1993). *Bootstrapping: A Nonparametric Approach to Statistical Inference.* Newbury Park, CA: Sage Publications.

Nelson, H. W. (1995). The relationship between volunteer long-term care ombudsmen and regulatory nursing home actions. *The Gerontologist, 35*, 509-514.

Nelson, H. W., Huber, R., & Walter, K. L. (1995). Long-term care volunteer roles on trial: Ombudsman effectiveness revisited. *Journal of Gerontological Social Work, 23*, 25-46.

Netting, E. F., Huber, R., Patton, R. N., & Kautz, J. R. (1995). Elder rights and the long-term care ombudsman program. *Social Work, 40*, 351-56.

Netting, E. F., Patton, R. N., & Huber, R. (1992). The long-term care ombudsman program: What does the complaint reporting system tell us? *The Gerontologist, 32*, 843-48.

Putnam, R. (2000). *Bowling Alone: The Collapse and Revival of American Community.* New York: Simon & Schuster.

Tocqueville, Alexis de. 1945. *Democracy in America.* New York: Knopf.

Verba, S., Schlozman, K. L., & Brady, H. E. (1995). *Voice and Equality: Civic Voluntarism in American Politics.* Cambridge, MA: Harvard University Press.

INNOVATION WITHIN ESTABLISHED FEDERAL-STATE PROGRAMS

Partnership Insurance: An Innovation to Meet Long-Term Care Financing Needs in an Era of Federal Minimalism

Mark R. Meiners, PhD
University of Maryland

Hunter L. McKay, PhD
U.S. Department of Health and Human Services

Kevin J. Mahoney, PhD
Boston College

SUMMARY. In the case of long-term care financing, federal minimalism is not new news. Long-term care has long played a weak "third fiddle" to national health reform concerns about the uninsured and catastrophic expenditures on prescription drugs. The states have been left to struggle with the issue of long-term financing as part of their responsibilities in

[Haworth co-indexing entry note]: "Partnership Insurance: An Innovation to Meet Long-Term Care Financing Needs in an Era of Federal Minimalism." Meiners, Mark R., Hunter L. McKay, and Kevin J. Mahoney. Co-published simultaneously in *Journal of Aging & Social Policy* (The Haworth Press, Inc.) Vol. 14, No. 3/4, 2002, pp. 75-93; and: *Devolution and Aging Policy* (ed: Francis G. Caro, and Robert Morris) The Haworth Press, Inc., 2002, pp. 75-93. Single or multiple copies of this article are available for a fee from The Haworth Document Delivery Service [1-800-HAWORTH, 9:00 a.m. - 5:00 p.m. (EST). E-mail address: getinfo@haworthpressinc.com].

10.1300/J031v14n03_05

funding and administering the means-tested Medicaid program. Recently, the environment has become even more challenging. Much of what is on the national agenda for health and welfare reform has been delegated to the states. This "devolution" of responsibilities has created many competing priorities for both the attention and resources of states.

This context of evolving federal minimalism calls for creative solutions that balance competing points of view. In this article, we provide some background and insights from one such effort: a collaboration between state governments and private insurers to put into operation an insurance-based approach to long-term care financing that uses Medicaid as an incentive to encourage potential purchasers. *[Article copies available for a fee from The Haworth Document Delivery Service: 1-800-HAWORTH. E-mail address: <getinfo@haworthpressinc.com> Website: <http://www.HaworthPress.com> © 2002 by The Haworth Press, Inc. All rights reserved.]*

KEYWORDS. Long-term care insurance, public-private partnership, state innovation, Medicaid, spend-down, nursing home, home care, asset protection

THE PROBLEM

Long-term care involves a broad array of supportive medical, personal, and social services needed by people unable to meet basic living needs due to illness or disability. Much of it is provided informally by family and friends. When care is purchased, the location typically involves various non-medical settings, including the home as well as community-based facilities. As a result, private insurers were very hesitant to sell coverage for long-term care, and the costs for such care became a significant cause of catastrophic expenses for seniors.

By the mid-1980s, the lack of adequate insurance funding for long-term care in the United States was beginning to receive national attention, and the fact that Medicare does not cover long-term care was beginning to be recognized. The major role of Medicaid in paying those bills once people became impoverished was alarming state governments. During that time, a private long-term care insurance market began to develop, but it was still in its infancy. First-generation private policies were being criticized for their numerous limitations and shortcomings (prior hospitalization requirements, lack of meaningful home- and community-based care benefits, eligibility based on medical necessity); consumer group reaction to private insurance was often negative. Nonetheless, states were becoming interested in this new source of financing for its potential to reduce the fiscal pressure on their Medicaid programs. Through task forces and study commissions, states began to look for ways to encourage improved products and support broader market development.

THE PARTNERSHIP FOR LONG-TERM CARE

The interests of the states in exploring ways to make private long-term care insurance more appealing and affordable to the public encouraged the Robert Wood Johnson Foundation (RWJF) to launch an initiative that provided planning grants to selected states that demonstrated a commitment to these goals (Merrill & Somers, 1989; Somers & Merrill, 1991). California, Connecticut, Indiana, Massachusetts, New Jersey, New York, Oregon, and Wisconsin received support to define and develop a public-private insurance partnership to pay for long-term care. With the help of the National Program Office, based at the University of Maryland Center on Aging, the states participating in the planning phase developed strategies to encourage the purchase of private insurance (Meiners, 1988; Meiners & McKay, 1989). The states recognized that to broaden the market for long-term care insurance it was important both to decrease the cost of the policies and to increase their quality. This is a special challenge, since increasing the quality of insurance policies generally increases the premium, which cuts down on the market.

Solving this cost-quality dilemma was at the heart of the strategies used by the four states that ultimately implemented their public-private partnerships (California-1994, Connecticut-1992, Indiana-1993, and New York-1993) (Meiners, 1993). The key incentive is a unique approach that allows people who purchase a state-certified long-term care insurance "Partnership" policy to get help from Medicaid without having to exhaust their assets.

Broadening the Market by Reducing the Financial Risk

While the states explored a variety of ideas on how to encourage the use of long-term care insurance to help their citizens avoid impoverishment, the basic approach was the same: Buy a state qualified insurance policy and get special asset protection (McCall, Knickman, & Bower, 1991). The quality/cost trade-off was handled by assuring that purchasers with less than comprehensive coverage could still be protected from impoverishment.

Normally, when a long-term care insurance policy runs out, policy-holders risk having to spend virtually all their savings before qualifying for Medicaid. In contrast, when a Partnership policy is exhausted, the policyholder is eligible for coverage under Medicaid without having to deplete previous savings. The details of the models differed from state to state. The most interesting difference was between New York and the three other states.

In New York, Partnership policies are required to pay three years of nursing home care, six years of home care, or some combination, after which all remaining assets are protected. A high priority of the New York approach is to offer middle- and upper-class seniors a viable alternative to giving away their assets and impoverishing themselves in order to qualify for Medicaid (Holubinka, 1992).

The underlying logic of this "total-assets" model is that the period of insurance is equal to or exceeds the time during which a person would be penalized by having to pay for long-term care if he or she had transferred assets in order to become eligible for Medicaid. When the program in New York began, this period was 30 months. Securing a three-year commitment to pay nursing home costs with private insurance would save the state money as compared to when someone is divested of his or her assets to receive Medicaid's assistance.

California, Connecticut, and Indiana adopted a "dollar-for-dollar" model. In addition to serving as an alternative to transferring, it allows people to buy a policy that protects a specified amount of their assets. An individual with $50,000 in assets might buy $50,000 in insurance protection while another individual with $150,000 in assets might buy $150,000 in insurance protection. Payments for long-term care by the insurance company are considered the equivalent of spending assets for the purpose of establishing Medicaid eligibility (Mahoney, 1992). Thus, a person who purchased a $75,000 policy would be able to keep $75,000 when he or she became eligible for Medicaid.

Though it would be simpler if all states used the same approach, both models have unique strengths. The total-assets approach provides the maximum incentive to purchase long-term care insurance (total-asset protection) and is arguably easier to understand because of its one-size-fits-all approach. It also fits better with existing long-term care insurance in that it requires at least three years of nursing home coverage. This had been the industry standard throughout much of the early market development. As such, the average commission per sale tends to be higher.

For insurers and agents, then, the total-assets model is often viewed as preferable to the dollar-for-dollar approach. They see it as the most reasonable compromise sale for those who cannot afford lifetime coverage, which is becoming the new industry standard sale.

The special strength of the "dollar-for-dollar" asset-protection model is that it makes purchases of insurance covering the equivalent of one to three years of benefits (e.g., anywhere from about $50,000 to $300,000, depending on the location) more meaningful by those in the middle to modest income group. Without the special asset protection, shorter, more affordable, coverage can still leave the purchaser at risk of impoverishment from catastrophic expenses. Faced with this possibility, people too often go without long-term care insurance, even though they need and could afford some protection.

In an interesting twist, Indiana revised its program to include a hybrid approach intended to get the best of both asset-protection strategies. Up to a set amount of coverage (the dollar equivalent of four years in the average Indiana nursing home) the purchaser is eligible for dollar-for-dollar asset protection while getting Medicaid benefits. But those who buy a policy covering more than this amount will receive total-asset protection along with help from Medicaid once they use up their insurance.

Quality Emphasis

The basic message of the Partnership emphasizes product quality–everyone should have some coverage, if necessary, trading lifetime less comprehensive coverage for shorter high-quality benefits–and then be able to access Medicaid's benefits without being impoverished if those benefits are not enough.

Each state's Partnership staff actively worked with Insurance Department analysts in reviewing and approving Partnership policies. In developing their approach to product quality, the states learned from and built on each other's experience. Connecticut was the first state to wrestle with the issue of standards (Mahoney & Wetle, 1992). Areas of agreement that emerged included the development of objective measures of functional and cognitive disability–rather than professional judgments regarding medical necessity–to determine when insurance coverage would be triggered; measuring cognitive impairment using observable behaviors; utilizing state-licensed independent care management agencies to develop care plans; and a commitment to create a uniform database documenting the use of service in an insured environment and preserving a record of the asset protection that each individual had accumulated (Spector, 1991; Mahoney, 1997).

The states that followed the dollar-for-dollar approach to asset protection built on one another's work in other respects as well. Indiana took Connecticut's approach to regulations and adapted them–mainly by standardizing benefit eligibility rules to assure greater continuity of coverage with Medicaid, if it was still needed after the insurance ran out. California, in turn, took Indiana's regulations and augmented them, insisting on numerous regulations for its participating insurers, all aimed at the special needs of consumers who had middle or modest incomes (Mahoney & Connolly, 1995; Mahoney et al., 1997). For example, California requires insurers to offer a one-year policy as a prerequisite to participation and has pioneered approaches (such as requiring state approval of initial premiums as well as rate increases) to prevent or mitigate premium increases and to prevent policy lapses.

New York took a different approach when it came to quality assurance. Rather than put new and higher standards into its regulations, the state put the special terms and conditions for the Partnership into contracts between the state and the insurers, a more flexible and less time-consuming approach (Nussbaum, 1992). New York relies on an "Evolution Board" that allows insurers and the state to share equal authority over major policy decisions. This arrangement cemented insurer support for the Partnership in New York and helped the state win special recognition for its efforts, including a 1995 Innovations Award in State and Local Government from the Ford Foundation and Harvard University's Kennedy School of Government.

Inflation protection–whereby the value of the policy rises by a specified percentage every year–is perhaps the best single example of the state's push for quality products. Lifetime coverage only assures avoidance of impoverishment if the product is inflation-protected and covers nursing home and home care. The states were especially concerned that without inflation protection a purchaser could end up impoverished from the deductible and co-payment responsibilities of a "lifetime" policy. For this reason, mandatory inflation protection is among the certification standards that insurers participating in the Partnerships must meet to help ensure that long-term care policies are of high quality.

Development of a Uniform Data System

One of the best examples of the partnership that emerged in this program is the uniform data system developed through the cooperative effort of the states, the insurers, the University of Maryland Center on Aging, and the program evaluator (Laguna Research Associates). Because of the interest and controversy surrounding the partnership concept, the participating states knew it was essential to require information from insurers with which they could monitor the program and the state's potential liability.

The states decided to capture detailed information at the individually insured level so that characteristics of persons purchasing insurance and utilizing benefits could be tracked. Person-level data help assure that information about asset protection will be available to insured persons and to the state if and when Medicaid contributed to a person's long-term care expenses.

During the implementation process, insurers realized that each of the four Partnership Programs intended to promulgate a unique set of requirements. The Health Insurance Association of America arranged a meeting at which it was strongly suggested that making the reporting requirements uniform would get more insurers to participate. Shortly after the meeting, the state Partnership Programs agreed that following through on the suggestion made by the insurers was important to the success of the partnership. This set in motion the creation of the uniform data set (UDS).

The development and maintenance of the UDS has been a challenge. Among the areas in which there were great differences were the fundamental purpose of the file, the willingness and ability of insurers to provide specific information, and state laws dealing with the release of individual-level data for research purposes. In spite of these differences in perspective, agreement was reached on a set of reporting requirements.

The data set has proven useful to the states and the Program Evaluator, providing information on the purchase and use of long-term care insurance benefits that is traditionally not available to the public. The following list shows some of the ways in which these data are currently being used:

- Transition Planning–When a Partnership policy holder is about to exhaust benefits, partnership staff can ensure that that beneficiary is aware of how the partnership works and, thus, gets the asset protection he or she is entitled to under the rules of the program.
- Product Sales–States are also using the UDS to ensure that the products being sold under the partnership license in fact do meet partnership standards. One of the states discovered a participating

insurer whose policy initially met the partnership licenser standards, but over time did not. The data set allows the states to identify and correct such problems.

- Research–The data set is used extensively by the Program Evaluator for research purposes. It provides data on the many aspects of the products that are sold under the partnership. Researchers thus have a common data set for four different states and can then supplement the baseline data with additional special studies.
- Policy Features–The Registry Files allow partnership staff to monitor the appeal of specific optional benefits, such as non-forfeiture, and provide information on its sale. States also have the option of monitoring how initial purchasers change their policies over time. This will allow for a calculation of lapse rates and of rate increases.

Unexpected Barriers to Program Implementation

The idea of the Partnership was hatched at a time when there was relatively little talk of universal health insurance. Participating states felt that the Partnership was an approach that would allow them to deal with long-term care in a helpful, budget-neutral way that could easily be supported. By linking the Partnership incentive to Medicaid, the constituency for the means-tested program could be enhanced rather than eroded (Meiners & McKay, 1990; Mahoney & Meiners, 1994; Meiners & Goss, 1994).

However, for advocacy groups such as AARP and Families USA, the means tested Medicaid was viewed as part of the problem that required a social insurance solution. The linking of long-term care insurance with Medicaid as a way to address financing problems of long-term care was philosophically unacceptable, if not damaging, to the case for a social insurance approach to long-term care.

Advocacy group opposition to the Partnership approach was far from unanimous. As the states worked to gain a consensus on key issues, it was not unusual for the local consumer representatives from groups such as AARP to end up in support of the Partnership in spite of the opposition from the national office. Local advocates liked the consciousness raising that went with the process of gaining acceptance of the enhanced standards of the Partnership.

While every RWJF Partnership was enacted as a result of unanimous votes in the state legislatures, the opposition at the federal level resulted in legislation that grandfathered the four RWJF State Partnerships but put restrictions on further replication. The Omnibus Budget Reconciliation Act of 1993 (OBRA '93) requires that any states implementing Partnership Programs after May 14, 1993, must recover assets from the estates of all persons receiving services under Medicaid. The result of this language is that, for replication states, the asset-protection component of the Partnership is still in effect but only while the insured is alive. After the policyholder dies, those states must recover what Medicaid spent from the estate, including protected assets.

OBRA '93 has had the effect of stifling interest in replicating the Partnership. Prior to passage of this legislation, interest in the Partnership had grown well beyond the four states funded by the Robert Wood Johnson Foundation. As many as 12 states had passed enabling legislation to create programs modeled on the Partnership. In recognition of the desire of states to deal with the long-term care financing problem, a bill (H. R. 1041) was recently offered that would eliminate the wording requiring estate recovery of protected assets and would remove the May 13, 1993, deadline for states to obtain an approved state plan amendment.

While the OBRA '93 restrictions were originally offered by a few key Democratic legislators who had reservations about private long-term care insurance, the reasons for not removing them today are more difficult to understand. There has been bipartisan support for long-term care insurance as a piece of the financing puzzle that culminated in the tax clarifications of HIPAA, and there has been serious talk of new premium credits as part of tax reform. One theory is that the political environment has changed so much since the Partnership Program began that the insurance industry is reluctant to support a compromise idea with the features of the Partnership Program.

Insurers and Agents as Key Partners

The program has represented a major change in the traditional relationship between state governments and insurers. Usually, contact is through the Department of Insurance, and then it has been mostly about issues related to product approvals and company solvency. The Partnership has involved a whole new layer of oversight. But when the program began, there was a strong sense on the part of key insurers that the market for long-term care insurance could benefit from the visibility and credibility brought about by working closely with state governments. Insurers and states were in agreement on the importance of private responsibility in paying for long-term care and the need to avoid dependence on Medicaid.

Initially, 22 insurers, accounting for the sale of three-quarters of the long-term care insurance policies sold nationwide, sought and received approval to market Partnership policies (McCall, Bauer, & Korb, 1996). Currently, the number of insurers participating is 30, with California being the most selective with 6 and Indiana being the most inclusive with 15. The insurers tend to participate in more than one state, but few are partners in all states. Nearly all insurers participating in the Partnership maintained their regular product offerings.

In all Partnership states, at least some insurers actively participated in the planning and implementation of product design, consumer education, and marketing. In-kind contributions toward printing and distribution of materials are common in the participating states, and several states have collected contributions toward general education and marketing activities.

Despite this support, the Partnerships found that their long-term care insurance package was not necessarily attractive to insurance agents. As the Partnership was implemented, insurers and agents voiced dissatisfaction with certain aspects of the program design:

- The program requirements deviated from some of the standard approaches used to market long-term care coverage and required extra attention. To get lifetime coverage within a limited budget often leads to dropping inflation protection. The Partnership strongly encourages shorter coverage that is inflation-protected as the preferred choice.
- Many insurance agents tend to avoid Medicaid, whose future they view as uncertain. Additionally, the Partnership model cannot be easily generalized because many state Medicaid programs do not offer comprehensive home and community benefits or systems of care management that characterize Partnership Programs. The participating states see Partnership insurance as both a public policy and market intervention that can help keep Medicaid viable for those who need it.
- The Partnership's policy development, approval process, data reporting, and other requirements have made some companies and agents reluctant to market Partnership policies because of the extra effort involved in participation. In contrast, the states see these efforts as a way to encourage high quality product sales of both Partnership and non-Partnership insurance. This gives policymakers the confidence to support educational campaigns that feature long-term care insurance as a reliable option to be seriously considered.

- The primary target audience for Partnership policies differs from the audience with which agents have customarily worked. Selling to the high end of the income and asset spectrum is easier than targeting sales to those of middle and modest means, who might benefit most from the Partnership product options. Moreover, agent commissions are directly related to the size of the premiums they sell. The states recognize this but see Partnership insurance as a way to broaden the market to include those more at risk of being impoverished from high long-term care costs. This group represents a much larger part of the market and is ripe for insurers and agents willing to go after those sales.
- The lack of portability of the Medicaid asset-protection feature if one moves to another state is yet another barrier to sales. While this has no effect on the value of the insurance benefit payment itself, it is a concern for those who might move and depend on the asset-protection feature as the primary motivation for choosing a Partnership policy. To address this concern, two Partnership states have recently accomplished a breakthrough remedy that can serve as an example for other states to follow. Indiana and Connecticut have passed legislation and received approval from the Center for Medicare and Medicaid Services (CMS, formerly known as HCFA) that allows for the portability of the Medicaid asset-protection benefit.

Assessment

Evaluating the Partnership is tricky business, fraught with technical challenges as well as various different perspectives of how to define success (Knickman, 2001). Much of what has been discussed so far in this article comes from the "continuous quality improvement" mindset that is associated with the kind of process evaluation done by program developers. From this perspective, problems are expected in the process of accomplishing success. As for the technical challenges of evaluating the Partnership Programs, issues of timing are especially noteworthy. The classic evaluation concern is whether the program had enough time for a mature assessment of its potential.

A case in point on the issue of evaluation timing is the recently published book on the Partnership (McCall, 2001). While very useful, a number of key analyses in the book were based on data that predated program adjustments that have had a significant effect on the market. For example, using data through 1996, Cohen compared the Partnership purchasers to a sample of non-Partnership purchasers in those same states, as well as to a national sample of purchasers (Cohen, 2001). He concluded that the Partnership Programs had not attracted the middle-income buyers it was targeting. But this assessment was heavily influenced by the New York data, the state with the largest sales during this early phase of the program. As noted above, New York had a target market somewhat different from the markets of other states.

Total Partnership policy applications grew from 28,000 in 1996 to 120,000 by the end of 2000. This significant boost can be attributed to two key factors. Over time, standards espoused by the Partnership plans have been applied to all policies–leading to comparable premiums for comparable products. Building on this, program redesigns in Connecticut (4th quarter 1996), Indiana (3rd quarter 1998), and California (4th quarter 1998) were undertaken to keep the programs current with non-Partnership product developments (Mahoney et al., 2001; Meiners, 2001). In each of these states, sales increased dramatically (in the range of 300%-500%, comparing one-year periods before and after the program adjustments) and the higher levels of sales are being maintained. The net effect is that many more policies are now being sold to the middle and modest income target market, and the target population assessment should be updated.

Some findings will not change with new data. All Partnership insurance is required to have inflation protection. When comparisons to non-Partnership insurance are made, this and other quality features will always be important points to consider in a careful assessment. Lower quality products purchased by those with modest resources are not a good buy just because they have lower prices. Market data on older sales may simply reflect nursing-home-only policies that were not inflation-protected. Inflation protection raises prices, and this issue was often avoided by insurance agents during policy sales in the early years of marketing long-term care insurance.

The Partnership states feel they are successful in providing quality coverage to persons of middle and modest means. This view received a welcome boost when, in the most recent review of long-term care insurance policies by *Consumer Reports* magazine, the Partnership Program received very positive treatment in a special side-bar article (*Consumer Reports*, 1997).

The evaluation complaint of too little time has an even more challenging dimension upon which both the Partnership evaluators and program developers agree. Only with policies in force for many years will we be able to make a reasonable assessment of savings to Medicaid because long-term care insurance involves substantial years of prefunding before claims are expected. In the meantime, the incremental effect of Partnership vs. non-Partnership insurance faces a constantly changing baseline with interactive influences that become difficult to sort out (Weiner, 2001).

Whereas it will be some time before significant numbers of clients have drawn on their benefits and an impartial evaluation of the cost-effectiveness of the Partnership approach can be undertaken, simulations have shown that this approach can be budget neutral (National Program Office, 1991). Also, two separate studies conducted by the outside evaluator have indicated that, overall, "The Partnership attracted beneficiaries who would not have purchased long-term care insurance if the Partnership did not exist" (McCall & Korb, 2001). Results from a more in-depth study in California show that, "Partnership policyholders had significantly smaller levels of income and assets than other purchasers of long-term care insurance during the time the Partnership policies were available. Even more surprising, their reported income and assets were smaller or about the same as the random sample (of potential California purchasers 55 to 75 years of age)" (McCall, 1997).

In some cases, the four state Partnerships seem to have started a movement toward industry-wide change; in other cases, the Partnerships seem to have been ahead of the times, or perhaps naive. And while the Partnerships can't claim full credit, they did play a key supportive role in developing several major innovations and qualitative improvements. These contributions include:

- *A new emphasis on inflation protection.* This feature clearly distinguishes Partnership from non-Partnership sales. But it also appears that the Partnerships may already be having an effect on non-Partnership sales as well. In California, when a long-term care insurance offering by the California Public Employees Retirement System copied the Partnership benefit structure and used Partnership-approved scenarios to describe the value of the compound inflation protection option, 65% of the buyers–nearly double the national average–bought this protection against inflation.
- *Catalyzing and augmenting efforts to improve private policies.* The Partnership movement stimulated and supported efforts to:

1. develop objective measures of functional and cognitive disability as determinants of the "insured event";
2. implement an approach for removing artificial restrictions so that a policy's full lifetime maximum benefit could be used in the community or the nursing home—wherever the consumer needed it to be used;
3. utilize and adapt care management approaches to tailor benefits to individual needs;
4. stabilize premiums by requiring state insurance department reviews of initial premiums and any requests for rate increases, mandating continuing actuarial review of reserves, and setting limits on future rate increases; and
5. prevent an unintentional lapse of coverage for those with cognitive impairments.

Focusing on the Future

The Partnership is now at the stage where revisions and refinements are being made to increase its market impact. State budgets are becoming the predominant source of financial support since grant funding from the Robert Wood Johnson Foundation has ended. In three of the four states, the Partnership has already been made a permanent part of the Medicaid program, with line-item budget support. California's Partnership has been extended to 2005, when it is expecting to seek similar permanent status.

While the introduction of tax-qualified plans brought about by the Health Insurance Protection and Portability Act (HIPPA) of 1996 has prompted renewed interest in the long-term care insurance market on the part of consumers, insurers, and states, there is a need to go further. The insurance industry favors tax credits that can be taken by anyone without income restrictions. If such tax breaks are politically possible, they will give the market a boost, but there is still a need to reach the moderate income and asset market targeted by the Partnership Program (Freudenheim, 1996). The incentive strategy used in the Partnership Program and the lessons learned about private insurance will be valuable as we seek to accomplish both private market and public policy goals.

Whether or not the Partnership Program is allowed to grow beyond the four states to further test what is possible remains to be seen. Insurance industry hesitance about pushing for repeal of the OBRA '93 restrictions creates a classic "catch 22" situation. Without the repeal of the

OBRA '93 restrictions, it may be difficult to stimulate the multi-state interest necessary to justify the commitment of resources by insurers to help the Partnership expand to meet its potential. The Partnership is clearly designed to balance the public interest with the need for a strong private market. It will be necessary for organizations like the National Governor's Association (NGA) to act on their call for elimination of federal barriers to public/private insurance partnerships like those in the RWJF states and for the expansion of authority to all states to implement such programs (National Governors Association, 1997). The NGA understands that states need and want the opportunity to explore options like the Partnership because they are faced with significant budget concerns about their Medicaid long-term care responsibilities.

Building on the lessons learned in the Partnership, ideas for next steps can be examined (Meiners, 1998). One line of thinking is to work with selected insurers and agents implementing a marketing approach specifically for potential buyers who have middle or modest means. Revisions of the Partnership and non-Partnership policies to make them more compatible have already helped broaden the market. Continuing such efforts will be important as new generations of insurance products emerge on the market.

Because state-by-state development is costly, the idea of a uniform national partnership has also prompted discussions among the states and the insurers who have been most active in the current Partnership effort. However, dependence on state Medicaid programs as the basis for the asset protection does not easily allow for reciprocity agreements between states, and insurance agents often find it easiest to sell their policies as an alternative to Medicaid.

Developing an asset-protection incentive strategy that is not linked to Medicaid is worth consideration. Removing the asset-protection incentive from its direct link to Medicaid could eliminate concerns about variations across states and over time in what Medicaid will cover. It might also serve to allow for some combination of income and assets to be protected. One approach to removing the asset-protection incentive from its direct link to Medicaid would be to create a new optional benefit in which states could choose to contribute to a backup funding pool (perhaps with federal matching funds like Medicaid's). Under this approach, there could be uniform benefits once a Partnership policy ran out.

An even more ambitious federal version of this approach could dramatically reverse the trend toward devolution to the states. A new voluntary option under Medicare could be created that would require the purchase of a certified private long-term care insurance policy in exchange for a commitment to protect some level of assets. An approach like this, modeled on the Partnership, was offered by Senators Kennedy and Wofford (1994) to supplement the long-term care proposals offered as part of the Clinton Health Reform plan (Kennedy & Wofford, 1994). This type of approach could be broadened to include the types of benefits covered by Medicare supplemental insurance, especially prescription drug costs, the other major source of catastrophic expenditures for senior and disabled citizens. It would provide dramatic relief to the states but would likely require some readjustments or trade-offs in responsibilities to balance the significant cost shift to the federal government.

CONCLUSION

With all the new responsibilities that have recently been devolved to states, one thing has not changed. There is a large untapped market of middle- and modest-income people who need help in preparing to pay for their long-term care. The Partnership for Long-Term Care offers a framework for a state-based strategy that builds incrementally on their current responsibilities. It offers real-world experience upon which to build an affordable way for states to offer this needed help.

The original goals of the Partnership Program center on giving consumers a viable way to pay for future long-term care costs by increasing the quality of long-term care insurance and making it affordable for middle-income individuals. The Partnership has a number of special features that should be viewed as appealing when all sides of the argument are considered. The program is fiscally conservative, helps middle-income people avoid impoverishment, serves as an alternative to Medicaid estate planning, promotes better quality insurance products, supports consumer protection efforts, enhances public awareness regarding long-term care needs and options, and helps maintain public support for the Medicaid program.

The Partnership has enjoyed persistent, patient support from states (Mahoney et al., 2001), insurers (Stucki, 2001), agents (Turner, Shelton, & Orr, 2001), consumers (Burns, 2001), and the Robert Wood Johnson Foundation (Somers, 2001)–the kind of support that comes when there is agreement that the problem needs to be solved, the program is promising, and everyone's collaboration is needed. The rationale that all participants could benefit from the Partnership has made it possible to go forward.

AUTHOR NOTES

Mark R. Meiners is Associate Professor, Department of Public and Community Health and Associate Director of the Center on Aging at the University of Maryland, College Park. He is Director of the Robert Wood Johnson Foundation Medicare/Medicaid Integration Program, an initiative to help states develop new systems of care that better coordinate acute, post-acute, and long-term care. He is also Director of the Robert Wood Johnson Foundation (RWJF) Partnership for Long-Term Care, an innovative state-based long-term care insurance program, and has led this initiative since its beginning in 1987. Dr. Meiners specializes in the areas of aging and health with emphasis on financing and reimbursement issues. Dr. Meiners is nationally recognized as one of the leading experts on financing and program development in long-term care.

Dr. Meiners can be contacted at the Center on Aging, Rm. 1240 HHP Building, College Park, MD 20742 (E-mail: mm56@umail.umd.edu).

Hunter L. McKay is currently Social Science Analyst at The U.S. Department of Health and Human Services, Office of the Assistant Secretary for Planning and Evaluation: Division of Aging and Long-Term Care Policy. Dr. McKay has worked for more than 15 years on Medicaid and health care issues from state government, insurer, and foundation perspectives. He specializes in long-term care, managed care, and aging policy. Dr. McKay served as the Deputy Director of the Robert Wood Johnson Foundation Partnership for Long-Term Care from 1988-1996.

Dr. McKay can be contacted at DHHS/ASPE, Room 424E, 200 Independence Ave., SW, Washington, DC 20201.

Kevin J. Mahoney is a faculty member at the Boston College Graduate School of Social Work where he serves as Associate Professor as well as National Program Director for the Cash and Counseling Demonstration and Evaluation, a policy-driven evaluation of one of the most unfettered forms of consumer direction of personal assistance services, funded by the Robert Wood Johnson Foundation and the Office of the Assistant Secretary for Planning and Evaluation at the U.S. Department of Health and Human Services. During his 28-year career in gerontology and long-term care, Dr. Mahoney has served in a number of policymaking and administrative positions in the state governments of Connecticut and California. Prior to coming to Boston College in 1999, he held academic appointments at Yale University, the University of Connecticut, the University of California-San Francisco and the University of Maryland.

Dr. Mahoney can be contacted at Boston College Graduate School of Social Work, Rm. 306 McGuinn Hall, Chestnut Hill, MA 02467 (E-mail: kevin.mahoney@bc.edu).

REFERENCES

Burns, B. (2001). Consumers. In N. McCall (Ed.), *Who Will Pay for Long-Term Care: Insights from the Partnership Programs* (pp. 125-148). Illinois: Health Administration Press.

Cohen, M. A. (2001). The partnership for long term care: The road ahead. In N. McCall (Ed.), *Who Will Pay for Long-Term Care: Insights from the Partnership Programs* (pp. 187-206). Illinois: Health Administration Press.

Consumer Reports. (1997). Long-term-care insurance special report. *Consumer Reports, 62*(10), 35-51.

Freudenheim, M. (1996, Nov. 17). Deductions coming for long-term care: Incentives to buy insurance may not entice many boomers. *New York Times.*

Holubinka, G. (1992). New York partnership for LTC insurance. *LTC News & Comment, 3*(2), 9-10.

Kennedy, E. M., & Wofford, H. (1994). Senate Bill 1833, 103d Congress, 2nd session, February 7.

Knickman, J. (2001). Introduction. In N. McCall (Ed.), *Who Will Pay for Long-Term Care: Insights from the Partnership Programs* (pp. xi-xvii). Illinois: Health Administration Press.

Mahoney, K. J. (1992). Financing long-term care with limited resources. *Journal of Aging and Social Policy, 4*(1-2), 35-50.

Mahoney, K. J. (1997). New models of long-term care insurance: New roles for care managers. *Geriatric Care Management Journal, 7*(3), 28-32.

Mahoney, K. J., & Connolly, L. (1995). Long-term care: California's trend-setting initiatives. *Compensation and Benefits Management, 11*(4), 7-13.

Mahoney, K. J., Guttchen, D., Phillips, D., Pierce-Mill, S., Hack, M. A., & Belardi, G. (2001). The states. In N. McCall (Ed.), *Who Will Pay for Long-Term Care: Insights from the Partnership Programs* (pp. 65-96). Illinois: Health Administration Press.

Mahoney, K. J., & Meiners, M. R. (1994). Private and social insurance–the feasible option. *The Western Journal of Medicine, 160*(1), 74-76.

Mahoney, K. J., Quinn, J., Geron, S. M., & Parker, M. (1997). Case management for private payers. In R. Newcomer & A. Wilkinson (Eds.), *Annual Review of Gerontology and Geriatrics, 1966: Focus on Managed Care and Quality Assurance,* 16, 140-161.

Mahoney, K. J., & Wetle, T. (1992). Public private partnerships: The Connecticut model for financing long-term care. *Journal of the American Geriatrics Society, 40*(10), 1026-30.

McCall, N. (1997). *How Partnership Purchasers Differ from Purchasers of Other Long-Term Care Insurance in California.* Laguna Research Associates, Health Policy Research Series, Discussion Paper #97-5.

McCall, N. (2001). *Who Will Pay for Long-Term Care: Insights from the Partnership Programs.* Illinois: Health Administration Press.

McCall, N., Bauer, B. J., & Korb, J. (1996). *Participation of Private Insurers in the Partnership for Long-Term Care.* Laguna Research Associates, Health Policy Research Series, Discussion Series Paper #96-5.

McCall, N., Knickman, J., & Bower, E. J. (1991). Public/private partnerships: A new approach to long-term care. *Health Affairs, 10*(1), 164-176.

McCall, N., & Korb, J. (2001). What have we learned from the Partnership for long-term care. In N. McCall (Ed.), *Who Will Pay for Long-Term Care: Insights from the Partnership Programs* (pp. 149-186). Illinois: Health Administration Press.

Meiners, M. R. (1988). Enhancing the market for private long-term care insurance. *Business and Health, 5*(7), 19-22.

Meiners, M. R. (1993). Paying for long term care without breaking the bank. *The Journal of American Health Policy, 3*(2), 44-48.

Meiners, M. R. (1998). Public-private partnerships in long-term care. In L. C. Walker, E. H. Bradley, & T. Wetle (Eds.), *Balancing Responsibilities for Financing Long Term Care: The Integration of Public and Private Roles* (pp. 115-133). Baltimore: The Johns Hopkins University Press.

Meiners, M. R. (2001). Reflections of a partnership insider on long term care financing. In N. McCall (Ed.), *Who Will Pay for Long-Term Care: Insights from the Partnership Programs* (pp. 289-302). Illinois: Health Administration Press.

Meiners, M. R., & Goss, S. C. (1994). Passing the "laugh test" for long-term care insurance partnerships. *Health Affairs, 13*(5), 225-228.

Meiners, M. R., & McKay, H. L. (1989). Developing public-private long-term care insurance partnerships. *Pride Institute Journal, 9*(4), 35-40.

Meiners, M. R., & McKay, H. L. (1990). Private versus social long-term care insurance: Beware the comparison. *Generations, 14*(2), 32-36.

Merrill, J. C., & Somers, S. A. (1989). Long-term care: The great debate on the wrong issue. *Inquiry, 26*(3), 317-320.

National Governors Association. (1997). Executive Committee, Winter Meeting Recommendations.

National Program Office (NPO). (1991). *RWJF's Long-Term Care Insurance Partnership Program: Cost-Effectiveness Estimates.* Technical Assistance Note, Robert Wood Johnson Foundation Program to Promote Long-Term Care Insurance for the Elderly. College Park, MD: University of Maryland Center on Aging.

Nussbaum, S. (1992). *The New York State Partnership for Long-Term Care.* The Bulletin–Official Publication of the New York City Association of Life Underwriters, *72*(2), 27-36.

Somers, S. A. (2001). The role of large foundations: To foster innovation. In N. McCall (Ed.), *Who Will Pay for Long-Term Care: Insights from the Partnership Programs* (pp. 283-288). Illinois: Health Administration Press.

Somers, S. A., & Merrill, J. C. (1991). Supporting states: Efforts to provide long-term care insurance. *Health Affairs, 10*(1), 177-179.

Spector, W. D. (1991). Cognitive impairment and disruptive behaviors among community-based elderly persons: Implications for targeting long-term care. *The Gerontologist, 31*(1), 51-59.

Stucki, B. R. (2001). Insurers. In N. McCall (Ed.), *Who Will Pay for Long-Term Care: Insights from the Partnership Programs* (pp. 97-112). Illinois: Health Administration Press.

Turner, P., Shelton, P., & Orr, T. (2001). Agents. In N. McCall (Ed.), *Who Will Pay for Long-Term Care: Insights from the Partnership Programs* (pp. 113-124). Illinois: Health Administration Press.

Weiner, J. M. (2001). The limits of the partnership for long-term care. In N. McCall (Ed.), *Who Will Pay for Long-Term Care: Insights from the Partnership Programs* (pp. 243-262). Illinois: Health Administration Press.

Implementation Issues for Consumer-Directed Programs: Comparing Views of Policy Experts, Consumers, and Representatives

Lori Simon-Rusinowitz, MPH, PhD
Lori N. Marks, PhD
Dawn M. Loughlin, PhD
Sharon M. Desmond, PhD
University of Maryland

Kevin J. Mahoney, PhD
Boston College

B. Lee Zacharias, MSW
The Zacharias Group

Marie R. Squillace, PhD
National Council on Aging

Ann Marie Allison, MA
Arthur Andersen

SUMMARY. An increasing number of aging community providers and consumers support consumer-direction (CD) in long-term care services. In regard to devolution, consumer-direction goes beyond the usual ap-

[Haworth co-indexing entry note]: "Implementation Issues for Consumer-Directed Programs: Comparing Views of Policy Experts, Consumers, and Representatives." Simon-Rusinowitz, Lori et al. Co-published simultaneously in *Journal of Aging & Social Policy* (The Haworth Press, Inc.) Vol. 14, No. 3/4, 2002, pp. 95-118; and: *Devolution and Aging Policy* (ed: Francis G. Caro, and Robert Morris) The Haworth Press, Inc., 2002, pp. 95-118. Single or multiple copies of this article are available for a fee from The Haworth Document Delivery Service [1-800-HAWORTH, 9:00 a.m. - 5:00 p.m. (EST). E-mail address: getinfo@haworthpressinc.com].

10.1300/J031v14n03_06

proach of shifting responsibilities from the federal government to state governments to bring programs "closer to the people." Consumer-direction goes even further by placing resources directly in the hands of consumers.

Yet, many questions remain unanswered regarding how to implement CD personal assistance services in general, and especially for older persons. This article describes the importance of examining views from multiple key stakeholders involved in implementing CD programs. We report on three background studies that have informed the Cash and Counseling Demonstration and Evaluation (CCDE) design and implementation–policy expert interviews as well as surveys and focus groups with consumers and representatives. As a fourth data source, we drew upon experiences in designing the CCDE and initial results from the first year of implementation. Each of the three studies on its own provided essential information for planning the CCDE. However, when we examined the studies together, and added CCDE design and implementation experiences, views expressed by the different stakeholders formed a type of multi-perspective "dialogue" that expanded our knowledge about implementing CD services. We hope this increased knowledge will help expand the availability of such services for consumers of any age who want to direct their own care. *[Article copies available for a fee from The Haworth Document Delivery Service: 1-800-HAWORTH. E-mail address: <getinfo@haworthpressinc.com> Website: <http://www.HaworthPress.com> © 2002 by The Haworth Press, Inc. All rights reserved.]*

KEYWORDS. Community-based long-term services, consumer-directed services, cash benefit

INTRODUCTION

I like being able to have a say in who . . . cares for me. (Elderly Arkansas consumer)

I would be able to hire somebody . . . and pay them. I like that. (New Jersey representative)

I feel a lot more comfortable with my friends helping me out. (Adult Arkansas consumer)

Most people want to have a say in matters that affect their daily lives. Elders and people with disabilities share this desire, especially when it comes to how and when they receive help with intimate personal care such as bathing, dressing, using the toilet, and preparing their meals. Yet, traditional programs that provide such help often lack a significant consumer-direction focus that allows or encourages consumers to be in charge of their services. This paper addresses issues in implementing consumer-directed services. Our goal is to expand our knowledge about this important topic by comparing the views of key stakeholders involved in consumer-directed (CD) programs (i.e., people having an interest in such programs). We hope that increased knowledge about implementing CD programs will help expand the availability of such services.

Consumer-direction for persons needing assistance with activities of daily living (ADLs) and other personal care tasks originated over two decades ago among younger persons with disabilities in the disability rights and independent living movements (DeJong, Batavia, & McKnew, 1992). More recently, the aging community began to adopt CD principles that maximize consumer choice and control when a coalition between the aging and younger disability communities emerged in the mid-1980s (Simon-Rusinowitz & Hofland, 1993; Ansello & Eustis, 1992). Interest in consumer choice expanded among some aging leaders in the early 1990s, in part due to a belief that CD care may lead to cost savings (Simon-Rusinowitz et al., 2000). For many years, people from the disability community have believed that having more control over their services would enable them to meet their needs and improve the quality of their lives for the same amount of money or less than required by traditional services. The Cash and Counseling Demonstration and Evaluation (CCDE) is a policy-driven evaluation of these beliefs. The CCDE is a test of one form of CD services–offering consumers a cash allowance and information services in lieu of agency-delivered services.

On a continuum of CD services offering differing levels of decision-making, control, and autonomy, a cash allowance is one of the more unrestricted forms of CD services (Stone, 2000). "Cash and Counseling" enables consumers to purchase services, assistive devices, or home modifications that best meet their needs. In principle, cash allowances maximize consumer choice and promote efficiency as consumers who shop for the most cost-effective providers may be able to purchase more services (Kapp, 1996). In regard to devolution, consumer-direction goes beyond the usual approach of shifting responsibilities from the federal government to state governments. Devolution to states is designed to bring programs "closer to the people" as states can be more responsive to individual needs than a more removed federal government. Consumer-direction goes even further by placing resources directly in the hands of consumers.

We need to know more about how this approach works. The CCDE, co-sponsored by The Robert Wood Johnson Foundation and the U.S. Department of Health and Human Services, Office of the Assistant Secretary for Planning and Evaluation, seeks to learn whether this approach can increase consumer choice and control costs by empowering persons with disabilities to purchase the assistance they need to be as independent as possible. This three-state social experiment is taking place in Arkansas, Florida, and New Jersey Medicaid programs under Section 1115 Research and Demonstration Waivers granted by the Centers for Medicare and Medicaid Services. Elders (over age 65) and adults (age 18-64) are included in all states. Children with developmental disabilities are included in Florida.

This article describes the importance of examining views from key stakeholders involved in implementing CD programs. We report on three studies that have informed the CCDE design and implementation. These studies included a variety of methodologies and distinct sample groups to assess diverse views from key stakeholders. As a fourth data source, we drew upon experiences in designing the CCDE and initial results from the first year of implementation. While these three studies and CCDE experience speak about a cash allowance, many issues that are addressed are applicable to other types of CD programs.

BACKGROUND

Implementing Consumer-Directed Programs

Consumer-directed programs that encourage maximum consumer choice and full participation in community activities are a shift in focus for programs serving older persons, which have traditionally been more paternalistic in nature and focused on a more limited goal of keeping older persons in their own homes and out of nursing homes. Increased choice and control is likely to increase satisfaction with care and quality of life (Ansello & Eustis, 1992; Doty, Kasper, & Litvak, 1996; Kapp, 1996; Simon-Rusinowitz & Hofland, 1993). Although an increasing number of aging community providers and consumers support more consumer control and choice within service delivery, many questions remain unanswered regarding how to implement CD personal assistance services (PAS) in general, and especially for older persons (Doty, Kasper, & Litvak, 1996; Kapp, 1996; Mahoney, Estes, & Heumann, 1986; Simon-Rusinowitz & Hofland, 1993). For example, researchers are exploring appropriate approaches to assessing consumers' preferences regarding their services and assuring high quality services in CD programs–critical implementation issues (Davis, Schneider, Kunkel, & Applebaum, 2001; Geron, 2000; Degenholtz, Kane, & Kivnick, 1997).

Views of Key Stakeholders Involved in Implementing CD Programs

Consumer-direction is an innovative approach that could challenge the way long-term care is delivered. While many service providers and consumers have been excited by CD, as with any system change, there has been resistance to the concept. For example, service providers who felt threatened about losing clients to the cash option were likely to express doubt about and resistance to this program. According to Green and Kreuter's health promotion planning model (1999), people will appreciate and support health innovations and policies if they can see clearly how such efforts address their concerns and contribute to the quality of their lives.

This model stresses the principle of participation to ensure the involvement of the people intended to benefit from a proposed program. Green and Kreuter (1999) describe a "social assessment" process that involves gathering information from multiple sources to expand the understanding of people regarding the quality of their own lives. They explain that lay people may view health from different perspectives than do professionals. Professionals tend to focus on the objective indicators of health, while lay people tend to emphasize subjective indicators such as social, emotional, spiritual, and cultural dimensions of health (Green & Kreuter, 1999). All perspectives are necessary for successful program planning. This principle was clearly demonstrated by the CCDE background research. The perspectives of policy experts as well as those of consumers and/or their representatives (relatives or friends), expressed in surveys and focus groups, guided program planners in designing the project. These varied perspectives were sometimes supportive of one another, while at other times there was tension among them.

The social assessment process includes two imperatives. The first is a pragmatic imperative: Joint participation is necessary when tackling today's complex health problems. Community members have insights and knowledge that professionals may not have. Also, community involvement may encourage community buy-in to program innovations. The second is a moral imperative: including community members in the planning process shows respect for potential program participants. Green and Kreuter (1999) emphasize the importance of planning *with* community members, rather than *for* communities. While Green and Kreuter's planning process has been applied extensively in the health promotion field, its application to an aging and disability social experiment is new to our knowledge.

The Key Stakeholders

To represent key stakeholders in designing CD services, we gathered information from multiple perspectives and used a variety of methodologies. First, we interviewed 20 policy experts from the aging and disability arenas. Participants included state program administrators and leaders in home- and community-based services from multiple settings. Next, we conducted focus groups and surveys with consumers and/or representatives in the Demonstration states who would be eligible to participate in the CCDE. The experts were able to contribute insights about the political and health care provider climate, and consumers/representatives added a dimension that enabled program planners to design a CD program that could serve them well. Views from additional stakeholders came from the fourth data source in this study, actual CCDE experiences in designing the Demonstration and first year implementation data. This source brings firsthand experiences of Demonstration state staff, policymakers, traditional personal care agencies, and the project management team (composed of the project funders, project directors, evaluation specialists, and others).

Various stakeholders had different roles in this process. Policy experts were asked to raise issues and concerns about implementing CD services, and speak about the perspectives of consumers, providers, payers, and policymakers. Thus, policy experts' comments represent their own views as well as predictions about these four constituencies. Consumers and representatives were asked to share their preferences about a CD cash option. Program planners then considered the information provided by these studies to find solutions to the concerns and preferences raised by policy experts, consumers, representatives, and others. These various roles illustrate how a "dialogue," or even some tension, among key stakeholders became part of the program planning and design process.

METHODS

Descriptions of the Three Studies[1]

Policy Expert Interviews. Telephone interviews were conducted with 20 policy experts from the aging and disability communities. The research questions were designed to assess implementation issues when adopting a CD approach to aging services and to address issues as they relate to consumers, providers, payers, and policymakers. Nine participants had experience specifically in aging issues; ten participants described working with both elders and younger persons with disabilities; and one participant had experience only with disability issues. Policy experts were affiliated with the federal government (2), state government (1), universities (7), other research settings (2), national associations (3), one private foundation, and one health insurance company. Three experts were private consultants. Interviews were conducted between September 1996 and August 1997. The interviews ranged in length from 25 to 125 minutes, and averaged 76 minutes. Refer to Simon-Rusinowitz et al., 2000, for a detailed description of the policy expert study.

Telephone Surveys. Surveys with consumers and representatives were conducted in Arkansas, New York,[2] New Jersey, and Florida. Medicaid personal care clients were randomly selected from the total Medicaid personal care clients in those states. The sample size and response rate for each state were: Arkansas (n = 491, 34%), New York (n = 493, 31%), New Jersey (n = 683, 60%), and Florida (n = 743, 50%).[3]

A 139-item instrument was developed to measure consumer and representative perceptions of a cash option. The survey assessed consumers' satisfaction with current PAS, perceptions about the cash option, and demographic and background variables, as well as representatives' perceptions and demographics. Telephone interviews took place between April and November 1997. On average, interviews lasted 40 minutes. If respondents felt unable to answer survey items themselves, they provided the interviewer with the name and phone number of a representative responder. Items were worded so it was very clear to representatives when they were answering for the consumer and when they were providing their own opinions. Refer to Simon-Rusinowitz et al., 1997; Mahoney et al., 1998; Mahoney et al., 2002; and Desmond et al., 2001 for detailed descriptions of the telephone surveys.

Focus Groups. Focus groups with consumers and representatives were conducted prior to the telephone surveys to guide survey development. In addition, a series of focus groups was conducted after the surveys to help explain survey findings.

Eleven focus groups with a total of 96 participants were conducted in Westchester County and New York City, NY, and in Tampa, FL, in late 1996 and early 1997. These groups were conducted to: determine consumer satisfaction with current Medicaid personal care, introduce the concept of the cash option, gauge consumer and representative reactions to the program features, determine consumer and representative reactions to the cash option tasks, and determine if there are certain demographic characteristics that affect one's desire to participate in the cash option. Focus group participants included adults with physical disabilities under age 65, elders over age 65, and representatives who assist in decision-making with consumers who are unable to make all decisions for themselves. A second series of 16 focus groups, with a total of 95 consumer and representative participants, was conducted after the telephone surveys to obtain further explanation of survey findings. Refer to Simon-Rusinowitz et al. (in progress) for a full discussion of focus group findings.

Implementation Data. Initial observations from CCDE planning activities and experience from the first year of implementation in Arkansas were considered in this study, including preliminary findings from a survey of early Arkansas consumers who had been in the cash option for nine months (Brown & Foster, 2000). Survey participants included 194 individuals who enrolled in the Arkansas demonstration between its inception (December 1998) and June 1999, were randomly assigned to receive the cash allowance, and completed a nine-month follow-up interview between September 1999 and March 2000. The telephone survey had a 90% response rate. It included descriptive information about cash option consumers and well as consumer outcomes in four areas: program participation; uses of cash, goods, and services; hiring of caregivers; and satisfaction.

Procedures for the Secondary Analysis

In this secondary analysis, we began by identifying and examining common themes expressed by different stakeholders across the data sources. (In this retrospective analysis, each data source did not necessarily address each topic discussed.) We noted that in many cases, policy experts and consumers had different perspectives about CD principles–exhibiting a tension between the differing perspectives. They expressed different views about whether consumers would be willing to participate in CD services, whether consumers would be able to manage CD services, and whether CD services could be successfully implemented.

Each of the three background studies on its own provided essential information for planning the CCDE. However, when we examined the studies together, and added CCDE design and implementation experiences, views expressed by the different stakeholders formed a type of multi-perspective "dialogue" about CD. In this dialogue, for instance, policy experts sometimes expressed concerns, and the issues about which they were concerned were then "resolved" by consumers and program planners during the often-challenging program development phase of the CCDE. At the same time, ideas for CD implementation were often expanded as a result of comparing views from the stakeholders.

FINDINGS

It's offering you the same options that you're getting. The only difference is that you're in charge. (Florida elder)

This section reports results from the four data sources that illustrate the need to compare multiple views among stakeholders regarding CD services. Policy experts, consumers and their representatives, and Demonstration staff expressed differing views about the topics discussed in this article. These contradictory views could have presented barriers in designing the CCDE had we not examined the responses of all involved. Stakeholders' concerns and eventual solutions to those concerns about consumers' ability to manage CD services, fraud and abuse, consumer training, and worker shortages are presented and summarized in Table 1.

Stakeholders' Concerns About Consumers' Ability to Manage CD Services

Experts were concerned about allowing individuals who could not manage CD tasks independently to participate in the CCDE. Although project implementers initially shared this concern, they decided that they did not want to exclude any individuals who could benefit from the program. Implementers looked for ways to be inclusive and decided to allow a surrogate or representative for individuals who need assistance with decision-making. The CCDE includes all consumers interested in the cash option, regardless of disability level, and allows representatives to assist consumers who cannot manage all consumer tasks independently.

Policy experts expressed further concerns about how to identify whether consumers can manage CD services because procedures to assess consumers' skills in managing CD services were not clearly defined. Their thoughtful statements illustrated this difficult issue. "There is also the question of how you determine the skill levels of the consumers in managing CD services. . . . " "An issue also is how you determine for whom CD services are appropriate and desired, and for whom they are not." Using a representative addresses these issues.

Policy experts, consumers, and representatives were concerned about the need to serve consumers with a variety of needs, preferences, and impairments. They discussed differences in the level of interest in CD, specifically the cash option, depending on consumers' demographic and background characteristics such as age. Experts pointed out that consumers evolve and their needs change; thus, there is a need for multiple, flexible programs (8).[4] "People evolve through their lives. They have different wants and needs . . . programs should reflect the ability to evolve."

Differences in Interest Level by Age Groups. Policy experts predicted that consumers and providers might be resistant to CD services for elders. Experts reported that payers and policymakers' paternalistic thinking has made it difficult for them to accept an independent living philosophy for elders who have a wide range of health care needs (17). One expert added, "The potential for a more unstable health care condition of older people has been the rationale [of policymakers] for using agencies rather than a CD approach."

Contrary to the view that elders would be uninterested in CD services, survey data revealed that a substantial proportion of elders over age 65–one-third to one-half–were interested in this approach to services. Many older focus group participants expressed interest in the cash option and felt they would have no problem handling the tasks. "I think it would be great . . . I would have the control over who was going to come into my home, and what they were going to do . . . ." (Florida elder). In addition, preliminary findings indicate that 73% (n = 194) of Arkansas CCDE participants were elderly (which mirrors Arkansas' eligible personal care population since about three-fourths of the participants are elderly) (Brown & Foster, 2000). This experience is consistent with an evaluation of the California In-Home Supportive Services, a CD program, in which more than half of the participants were elderly (Benjamin & Matthias, 2001; Doty et al., 1999).

TABLE 1. Implementation Issues for Consumer-Directed PAS Programs: Comparing Stakeholders' Views and Experiences. Background Research to Support the Cash and Counseling Demonstration and Evaluation

Summary of Findings

Key Issues	Policy Expert Views	Consumer/Representative Survey Results	Consumer/Representative Focus Group Results	Experiences in CD Programs
Concerns about consumers' ability to manage CD services and the need for flexible programs to meet diverse consumers' preferences.	• Concerned about excluding individuals who could not manage CD tasks. • Predicted that older consumers may not want CD services. • Expressed need for flexible programs to include diverse consumers.	• One-third to one-half of elders were interested in CD approach. • African American and Hispanic consumers were more interested in C&C than were Caucasians.	• Many older participants expressed interest and felt they would have no problem handling tasks. • African American and Hispanic participants felt their cultures have strong family networks and emphasize caring for family members.	C&C Experience: • Created role of a representative for consumers needing help with employer tasks. • Preliminary findings show that 73% of AR C&C Demonstration consumers are elderly. • Consumers who knew someone to hire as a worker have done best in the cash option. Finding a worker may be easier in a community with strong family networks. CA IHSS Experience (Doty et al., 1999): • Over half of consumers in the evaluation were elders (over 65).
Concerns about family decisions truly representing consumers accurately.	• Concerned that family decision-making may not represent consumer accurately.	• A family member or friend completed the survey for 17% of consumers. • Representatives were able to differentiate between their views and views of consumers.	• One focus group respondent stated that she would "change her mother's mind" in order to convince her mother to agree with her daughter's choices.	• The nine-month CCDE report shows that about half of AR participants are represented by family or friends. • This issue needs to be studied further.

TABLE 1 (continued)

Key Issues	Policy Expert Views	Consumer/Representative Survey Results	Consumer/Representative Focus Group Results	Experiences in CD Programs
Concerns about fraud and abuse.	• Concerned that consumers unable to manage tasks could be vulnerable to fraud, abuse, and neglect. • Providers fear liability based on bad decisions made by consumers. • Concerned that even rare cases of fraud/abuse could cause bad publicity.	• Respondents were aware of cash option challenges and most (3/4) stated they would want training and/or assistance with employer tasks.	• Some felt they could handle employer tasks, others were interested in training or assistance.	• Early implementation experience in AR shows that fears of fraud and abuse were unwarranted. • CA IHSS (Doty et al., 1999) evaluation generally supports this experience.
Concerns about level and type of training needed.	• While some believed that training is important, some were concerned that too much training could make a CD program seem overly complicated.	• Most consumers/representatives (80%) said they would like a fiscal intermediary (FI) to help handle book-keeping tasks.	• Participants were willing to be trained or assisted with tasks. • Some saw contact with peers as a means to problem solving.	"Almost all AR consumers have used an FI to handle book-keeping tasks.
Concerns about worker shortages.	• Concerns about availability of trained service providers, quality of care, and obtaining backup services.	• Consumers and representatives also acknowledge need for help in finding workers and backup workers. • Respondents wanted to pay their workers more than agency wages.	• Respondents wanted to pay their workers more than agency wages.	"In AR, 78% of cash option paid workers are relatives. In the CA IHSS evaluation, almost half of the paid workers in the CD model were relatives and about a quarter were friends/ neighbors.

On the other hand, focus group discussions provided an explanation of why some older consumers were not interested in the cash option. For example, older consumers may not have been as interested initially as younger consumers since older consumers reported being more satisfied with current PAS than younger consumers. Many believe PAS enables them to remain in their homes. "I couldn't live in my apartment if I didn't have a homemaker," stated one Florida elder. A New York representative demonstrated the centrality of this desire for elders to be able to remain in their homes by saying, "The best thing about it (the cash option) is being able to keep your loved ones . . . in their own surroundings."

The focus groups revealed a possible explanation for the higher rate of younger consumer interest in the cash option. Younger consumers sometimes see PAS operating for agency convenience, not consumer needs. As one Florida consumer under age 65 stated, "Most nursing agencies want you to be home every day. Homebound you can't go to school. . . . So if you're trying to advance yourself . . . the system is really working against you. . . ."

Differences in Interest Level by Ethnic/Racial Groups. Following up on experts' statements about the need for flexibility in PAS to include all interested consumers, survey data revealed ethnic and racial differences in consumers' levels of interest in CD programs. According to survey data, African American and Hispanic consumers were more interested in the cash option than were Caucasians. Multivariate analyses demonstrated that consumers' race/ethnicity predicted their interest in the cash option in Arkansas, New Jersey, and New York. Focus group participants offered preliminary explanations of why African American and Hispanic consumers were more interested in the cash option than were Caucasians. African American and Hispanic participants felt their cultures tend to have stronger family networks and emphasize caring for family members. ". . . They are more caring. They got that family value . . . when it comes to sticking together, mostly they are really tight" (New Jersey African American representative).

Some believed that the cash option could bring much-needed jobs (as PAS workers) to African American and Hispanic communities. "It would be an income for someone else . . . some want to work and really need to work and can't get a job simply because they are African American and not a graduate or college student . . . " added an African American representative in Arkansas. Experience in Arkansas indicates slightly higher participation among African Americans than expected from the racial composition of the eligible personal care client population.

Concerns About Family Decisions Truly Representing Consumers

Experts pointed out that family members' participation in managing CD services could raise questions about the extent to which the consumer is actually directing the care. This issue was seen as a barrier to implementing CD services (7). "The preference and plans made . . . by any family member on behalf of the person with the disability might not be what they want." "A barrier is . . . disagreements . . . within families." Background research results and early CCDE implementation reports show that a significant proportion of consumers had representatives who completed their surveys (17%, n = 2140 in background research, and 50%, n = 194 in early CCDE implementation findings), demonstrating that this could be an important concern. Survey results indicate that representatives often expressed different views when speaking for consumers vs. when speaking for themselves, indicating that they were able to differentiate between their own views and the views of consumers. To the contrary, one focus group respondent stated that she would "change her mother's mind" in order to convince her mother to agree with her caregiving daughter.

Concerns About Fraud and Abuse

Policy experts were also concerned that consumers would not be able to handle CD tasks and therefore could be vulnerable to fraud and abuse. Experts reported that providers fear they may be liable for bad decisions made by consumers directing their own care (4). ". . . Agencies didn't want to provide services to people . . . because they were afraid that if the worker didn't show up that the person would be at risk. Then, the agency would be at risk." In addition, the New Jersey CCDE manager reported this issue as a major concern expressed when training consultants to assist consumers.

Experts also discussed payers' fears about client safety. They fear that people will be taken advantage of or be neglected. Experts predicted that payers and policymakers might resist implementing CD programs due to these fears about client and provider safety (11). "Even if fraud and abuse are very rare, one single case can cause so much damage. . . ." They added, "States need to think through . . . how to ensure quality . . . [policymakers] also don't want to be [in the headlines] with a scandal." The New Jersey CCDE manager's experience presenting this new program option throughout the state also illustrates the extent of this concern. His often-repeated experience was, "I say cash, they say fraud."

Experts reported that payers and policymakers also have concerns about accountability for cash payments and legal liabilities associated with CD programs (21). Among these concerns, "Payers will be concerned with . . . how the money is spent." One expert added, "[Payers] want to reduce administrative involvement but . . . they don't want to let go of the strings."

Experts were also concerned about whether consumers would pay their workers' taxes. They believed that consumers are limited in their knowledge of how to be an employer (19). "You have to take on this consumer role . . . in a time of great stress and impaired capacity." Thus, "Consumers [need] training [in] how to manage services [and] deal with the tax and liability issues."

Experts also warned that consumers should be aware of their vulnerability and need to be willing to assume the risks associated with managing their own care (6). "When you assume personal responsibility you also have to assume risk and that gets into who is liable for problems that may occur."

Survey data show that both consumers and representatives interested in the cash option system seem to be aware of the challenges and potential difficulty in those tasks. In all four states surveyed, more than three-fourths of consumers and representatives interested in the cash option stated that they would want training or help with payroll taxes, deciding how much to pay a worker, and doing a background check on the worker. Consumers' and representatives' strong desire for help or training demonstrates their willingness to handle consumer tasks appropriately.

First-year implementation data from Arkansas demonstrate that these fears of fraud and abuse are exaggerated. The majority of consumers have representatives and use fiscal intermediaries. There have been no reported cases of fraud and abuse. There was one instance of consumer self-neglect and that was addressed by requiring a representative for the consumer. Consumers report satisfaction with their services–93% stated they would recommend the program to others, and 82% reported that the cash option has improved their lives. None considered themselves to be worse off. The Arkansas experience is consistent with findings from an evaluation of the California In-Home Supportive Services program (IHSS), which reported that consumers in a CD program had higher ratings of client satisfaction, empowerment, and quality of life than consumers receiving traditional services (Doty, Benjamin, Mathias, & Franke, 1999).

Concerns About Level and Type of Training Needed

Stakeholders suggested that consumer training could address concerns about fraud and abuse, including liability for payroll taxes and misuse of the cash benefit. Most (80%) survey respondents said they would like to use a fiscal intermediary to help in handling payroll taxes, and would like training and support to help decide on pay, conduct background checks on workers, and interview workers.

Focus group findings added further support to survey results about consumers' and representatives' willingness to seek assistance with CD tasks. Participants had some concerns about finding and interviewing workers. Handling payroll tasks elicited the greatest concern and widest range of reactions. Participants with financial experience thought they could do payroll tasks with no training. One Florida participant stated, "I never worked outside the home, but I handled the money . . . I'm very interested in it (the cash option)." Those who were unsure about their abilities to handle payroll tasks willingly expressed their desire for training and support.

Experts speculated that too much training could be a barrier to implementing CD. In addition to the cost of training, one expert stated, "We could kill [this movement] by making it feel complicated, by suggesting that you have to have some sort of an advanced course in personal management. That you need to know so many things."

Concerns About Worker Shortages

Experts reported that in a CD program, consumers and providers often have concerns about the availability of trained service providers and obtaining emergency backup services. Experts predicted that this would also be a concern in the independent provider setting (2). ". . . We are wrestling with a shortage of backups and the nonexistence of a pool of capable personal assistants."

Another potential barrier to the availability of competent personal assistants is that independent providers have unique implementation issues such as being responsible for their own working conditions, adequate wages, benefits, and job security (8). "It's interesting about all the workers' issues coming up around CD . . . I think a lot of [agencies] use on-call labor pools who are poorly paid and get no benefits and are construed as working for themselves."

Experts pointed out that independent providers might find it difficult to coordinate the employment and tax regulations of the multiple programs in which an individual might participate (4). "Trying to coordinate [program rules] with a multi-problem individual who might cross over many programs . . . the providers might feel that they are at risk if they do things around CD rather than the regulation that the payer defined."

Surveys revealed that most consumers and representatives also acknowledge a need for help in finding workers and emergency backup workers. In fact, worker shortages have created difficulties in all three Demonstration states. Both surveys and focus groups showed that respondents wanted to pay their workers more. Consumers interested in the cash option were significantly more likely than those uninterested in the cash option to consider being able to pay their worker more money an important program feature.

DISCUSSION AND RECOMMENDATIONS

This section reviews new ideas about implementing CD services learned from the various perspectives reported in this study and makes recommendations about implementing CD programs.

Views from Multiple Stakeholders

The process of considering differing views from a variety of stakeholders resulted in a creative solution addressing concerns about consumers' abilities to manage CD services. Policy experts raised issues about identifying those consumers capable of managing CD services and focused on screening out consumers not able to be self-directing. CCDE program designers, in efforts to develop a solution to these potential problems, also acknowledged these issues. Their concerns were threefold: they did not want to exclude consumers who wanted to try a CD program; they were under pressure to meet enrollment requirements for the Demonstration; and they were worried about burdensome appeals/lawsuits from consumers who were told they could not participate. Hence, they chose an approach that would include all consumers, regardless of their abilities to be completely self-directing–the use of representatives. While this concept has been accepted in the developmental disabilities community for many years, it is new to CD programs and the aging community.

Investigate Messages to Change Attitudes of Some Stakeholders

Despite findings that many elders are interested in CD and are managing CD services, some stakeholders maintain their beliefs that elders are not interested in or capable of managing a CD program (Benjamin & Matthias, 2001; Brown & Foster, 2000; Mahoney et al., 2002). In designing their outreach and enrollment programs, the CCDE states have had to consider these beliefs about elders when determining who would be most effective in outreach and enrollment efforts. As previously mentioned, CD programs for elders are fairly new, and acceptance of this approach requires a paradigmatic shift from thinking about elders in a traditional, paternalistic manner (i.e., elders are frail and need to be taken care of) to being open to the possibility that some elders and their representatives may be interested in the choice and autonomy offered by a CD program. Clearly, it will be important to select outreach workers who are open to this concept for all consumers, including elders.

Stakeholders' concerns about fraud and abuse have been cited as another barrier to implementing CD programs. Information from the multiple data sources revealed many solutions or "antidotes" to consumer fraud and abuse. In response to policy experts' concerns, several CCDE features (i.e., training, representatives, and fiscal intermediaries) were designed to help deter fraud and abuse. Early implementation experience in Arkansas demonstrates that widespread fraud and abuse have not materialized. Survey and focus group data indicated that the majority of consumers and representatives were interested in and willing to participate in training to learn necessary employer skills and planned to utilize a fiscal intermediary service for payroll tasks. Representatives provide support for the most vulnerable consumers who are unable to manage all employer tasks independently; training empowers consumers and representatives with needed skills; and the fiscal intermediary limits the amount of cash in consumers' hands, while assuring that employer and employee taxes will be paid. In addition, all consumers, including those with representatives, are monitored by CCDE consultants.

CCDE as One Solution to a Shortage of Qualified PAS Workers

Policy experts, state CCDE staff, and consumers and representatives have all expressed concerns about the shortage of qualified PAS workers in an economy with low unemployment. This labor shortage is creating problems for agencies and consumers who try to hire independent workers. The perspectives from different stakeholders about this issue have led to several key social marketing messages that present the cash option as one approach to addressing the worker shortage.

First, survey and focus group data indicated that consumers and representatives are attracted to the idea that they can pay their workers more than they receive while employed by agencies. Consumers and representatives were acutely aware of the difficulty of finding and keeping good workers, and wanted to be able to pay competitive wages.

Second, consumers are likely to be attracted to the idea that they may receive services sooner in the cash option than in traditional services, especially if they are in a location that is difficult to serve. Agencies are not always able to serve their consumers immediately due to the worker shortage, especially those in rural areas who require much travel time for staff.

Home care agencies are important stakeholders in the CCDE, and state CCDE staff have worked to gain cooperation from these agencies. As predicted by policy experts and state CCDE staff, home care agencies initially viewed the cash option as a threat to their businesses. Yet, agencies were having difficulty serving clients due to labor shortages. Consequently, they have responded positively to marketing messages that encourage them to refer "hard to serve" consumers to the cash option. Consumers may be difficult to serve for a number of reasons (e.g., location, need for evening and weekend hours not usually offered by agencies), and these consumers may have their needs met in a more satisfactory manner by hiring workers independently.

Hiring consumers' relatives and friends as PAS workers is a way to expand the worker supply as this approach taps new worker sources who may not have entered the PAS labor force. Many of these new PAS workers will provide personal care for a family member out of devotion and caring, but would not have otherwise done so. Early findings about cash option participants in Arkansas indicated that the majority of consumers (78%) have hired relatives as paid workers; 15% hired a friend, neighbor, or church member; and few have hired strangers. There is also the possibility that paid relatives and friends will find this work satisfying and continue in the workforce when their relatives/friends no longer need their services. This approach to expanding the PAS worker labor force is potentially attractive to agencies, program administrators, and policymakers.

Ethnic/Racial Differences in Interest in Consumer-Directed Programs

The policy experts clearly stated the need to design programs flexible enough to meet the needs of diverse consumers. (They were not asked to comment on differing levels of interest in CD by racial/ethnic groups, and no experts raised this issue.) The telephone surveys revealed that African American and Hispanic consumers and representatives were more interested in the cash option than Caucasian consumers. In follow-up focus groups, African American and Hispanic consumers and representatives indicated that their cultures tend to have strong family networks that emphasize caring for one another. It is reasonable to conclude that consumers from closely-knit families and communities would have an easier time than consumers with fewer connections in achieving the first, critical step in a CD program–locating and hiring a worker. Thus, the strong networks of African American and Hispanic consumers may contribute to their increased interest in the cash option. Yet, the experience in Arkansas indicates only slightly higher participation among African American consumers than expected from the racial composition of the eligible personal care population, and less than expected based on preference study findings. We need to learn more about this issue.

Appropriate Levels of Consumer/Representative Training

Stakeholders were concerned about offering appropriate levels of training for consumers and representatives. Determining the "right" amount of training requires balancing the need to teach CD skills (i.e., performing employer tasks) with the need to keep the program manageable. As policy experts astutely indicated, making the program feel overcomplicated could kill it. Yet, the temptation to teach consumers and representatives as much as possible is great since consumer training is an important "antidote" to the major fraud and abuse concerns expressed by policymakers, program administrators, and others.

Recent focus groups with Florida case managers demonstrated some difficulties that occur when a program seems complicated. While they were complimentary about Florida's training materials, consultants thought the program was complicated and required a great deal of time to learn. As they felt burdened by their existing caseloads, they were overwhelmed at the prospect of learning a new program option that would add to their responsibilities. The case managers believed that consumers, particularly frail elders, would be overwhelmed by the program. These training issues need further attention.

Conclusion and Research Recommendations

Investigating the views of key stakeholders has revealed significant implementation issues for conducting CD programs, in general, and specifically cash allowance programs, and at least three areas for further research. This study has emphasized the need for investigating the role of representatives in CD programs, ethnic/racial differences in consumers' interest in CD, and effective training for consumers, representatives, and consultants. First, we need to understand better the role of representatives and examine whether they are truly representing consumers. How do representatives learn their role? How is the effectiveness of this role assessed? These questions have implications for numerous aspects of program design and evaluation, including training programs for participants and quality assurance priorities. A program cannot be truly consumer-directed unless representatives are eliciting consumers' views.

Second, we are just beginning to learn about the role of race and ethnicity in preferences for CD programs. Finally, in regard to training, we need to learn more about behavior-change efforts in regard to helping some professionals achieve a paradigm shift from a focus on dependency in a traditional home care model to a focus on consumer empowerment in a CD model. We also need to learn more about effective training for consumers and consultants to teach necessary skills while avoiding an overly complicated program. We look forward to learning more about these important issues as the CCDE continues and in follow-up research.

NOTES

1. The three studies are described in detail in reports and publications from each project. Interested readers can refer to the citations in this section to identify individual reports/publications.

2. New York was a Demonstration state early in the CCDE.

3. This survey consisted of Florida elders (age 65 and older) and adults with physical disabilities (age 18-64 years). Adults and children with developmental disabilities were surveyed separately.

4. The number in parentheses indicates the number of statements related to each topic addressed by the experts. Not all experts commented on each topic; however,

some experts provided multiple, distinct comments related to a topic. Thus, the number of comments may exceed the number of experts interviewed (20).

AUTHOR NOTES

Lori Simon-Rusinowitz is Deputy Director of the Cash and Counseling Demonstration and Evaluation (CCDE) at the University of Maryland Center on Aging and a faculty member in the Department of Public and Community Health. Her research focus has been in the field of aging and disability policy issues for the past 15 years. As Director of Research for the CCDE, Dr. Simon-Rusinowitz has overseen a three-part study of consumers' preferences for consumer-directed personal care as well as other components of the Demonstration and Evaluation.

Dr. Simon-Rusinowitz can be contacted at National Program Office, University of Maryland Center on Aging, HHP Building, College Park, MD 20742 (E-mail: ls119@umail.umd.edu).

Lori N. Marks is an adjunct faculty member for the University of Maryland, Department of Family Studies, and serves as a research consultant for the Cash and Counseling Demonstration and Evaluation.

Dr. Marks can be contacted at 9905 DePaul, Bethesda, MD 20817.

Dawn M. Loughlin has been involved in research design and program development in the fields of health and health policy since 1987–as a developmental psychologist, counseling program developer, and statistical analyst. She is currently a faculty research assistant with the University of Maryland, Center on Aging.

Dr. Loughlin can be contacted at National Program Office, University of Maryland Center on Aging, HHP Building, College Park, MD 20742.

Sharon M. Desmond is Associate Professor in the Department of Public and Community Health at the University of Maryland. She has participated in the Cash and Counseling Demonstration and Evaluation preference study survey team since 1997.

Dr. Desmond can be contacted at the Department of Public and Community Health, University of Maryland, College Park, MD 20742.

Kevin J. Mahoney is a faculty member at the Boston College Graduate School of Social Work where he serves as Associate Professor as well as National Program Director for the Cash and Counseling Demonstration and Evaluation, a policy-driven evaluation of one of the most unfettered forms of consumer direction of personal assistance services. During his 28-year career in gerontology and long-term care, Dr. Mahoney has served in a number of policymaking and administrative positions in the state governments of Connecticut and California. Prior to coming to Boston College in 1999, he held academic appointments at Yale University, the University of Connecticut, the University of California-San Francisco and the University of Maryland.

Dr. Mahoney can be contacted at Boston College School of Social Work, McGuinn Hall 132, Chestnut Hill, MA 02467.

B. Lee Zacharias is President of the Zacharias Group. She has moderated and written reports for most of the focus groups conducted for the Cash and Counseling Demonstration and Evaluation.

Ms. Zacharias can be contacted at 441 N. Pownal Rd., New Gloucester, ME 04260.

Marie R. Squillace is Senior Researcher for the National Council on the Aging. Her research has focused primarily on health and long-term care issues with specific interest in long-term care financing and organization. Most recently, Dr. Squillace is involved in efforts to transfer models of consumer-direction from the disability arena into the aging service system and in exploratory research to understand and gauge interest in approaches to consumer-direction in managed care.

Dr. Squillace can be contacted at Mariners Cove, 308 I Forbes St., Annapolis, MD 21401.

Ann Marie Allison obtained her master's degree from the University of Maryland in Career Counseling, Education, and Personnal Services. She worked with the Cash and Counseling Demonstration and Evaluation as a graduate assistant when she was a master's degree student. Since graduating, Ms. Allison has been working in various areas of organizational development as a manager in Human Resources at Arthur Andersen.

Ms. Allison can be contacted at 4845 Chevy Chase Drive, Chevy Chase, MD 20815.

REFERENCES

Ansello, E., & Eustis, N. (1992). A common stake? Investigating the emerging intersection of aging and disabilities. *Generations, 16*, 5-8.

Benjamin, A. E., & Matthias, R. E. (2001). Age, consumer direction, and outcomes of supportive services at home. *The Gerontologist, 41*(5), 632-642.

Brown, R., & Foster, L. (2000). Cash and counseling: Early experiences in Arkansas. Mathematica Policy Research, Inc., Issue Brief, Dec., No. 1. Princeton, NJ.

Davis, S., Schneider, B., Kunkel, S., & Applebaum, R. (2001). Quality monitoring in consumer directed care programs. Draft. Scripps Gerontology Center, Miami University, Oxford, OH.

Degenholtz, H., Kane, R. A., & Kivnick, H. Q. (1997). Care-related preferences and values of elderly community-based LTC consumers: Can case managers learn what's important to clients? *The Gerontologist, 37*(6), 767-776.

DeJong, G., Batavia A., McKnew, L. (1992). The independent living model of personal assistance in national long-term care policy. *Generations, 16*, 89-95.

Desmond, S. M., Mahoney, K. J., Simon-Rusinowitz, L., Shoop, D. M., Squillace, M. R., & Fay, R. A. (2001). Consumer preferences for a consumer directed cash option versus traditional services. Telephone survey findings of Florida elders and adults with physical disabilities. *Elder's Advisor, 3*(1), 1-22.

Doty, P., Benjamin, A. E., Matthias, R. E., & Franke, T. M. (1999). In-Home Supportive Services for the Elderly and Disabled: A Comparison of Client-Directed and Professional Management Models of Service Delivery. USDHHS Office of the Assistant Secretary for Planning and Evaluation, Contract #100-94-0022.

Doty, P., Kasper, J., & Litvak, S. (1996). Consumer-directed models of personal care: Lessons from Medicaid. *Milbank Memorial Fund, 74*(3), 377-409.

Geron, S. M. (2000). The quality of consumer-directed long-term care. *Generations, 24*(3), 66-73.

Green, L. W., & Kreuter, M. W. (1999). *Health Promotion Planning: An Educational and Ecological Approach.* Third Edition. Mountain View, CA: Mayfield Publishing Company.

Kapp, M. (1996). Enhancing autonomy and choice in selecting and directing long-term care services. *The Elder Law Journal, 4*(1), 55-97.

Mahoney, C., Estes, C., & Heumann, J. (Eds.) (1986). *Toward a Unified Agenda: Proceedings of a National Conference on Disability and Aging.* San Francisco: University of California and World Institute on Disability.

Mahoney, K. J., Desmond, S. M., Simon-Rusinowitz, L., Shoop, D. M., Squillace, M. R., & Fay, R. A. (2001). Consumer preferences for a consumer directed cash option versus traditional services. Telephone survey findings of New Jersey elders and adults with disabilities. In press, *Journal of Disability Policy Studies*.

Mahoney, K. J., Simon-Rusinowitz, L., Desmond, S. M., Shoop, D. M., Squillace, M. R., & Fay, R. A. (1998). Determining consumers' preferences for a cash option: New York telephone survey results. *American Rehabilitation*. 24(4) 24-36.

Mahoney, K. J., Simon-Rusinowitz, L., Loughlin, D. M., Desmond, S. M., & Squillace, M. R. (2002). Determining personal care consumers' preferences for a consumer-directed "Cash and Carry" option: Survey results from Arkansas, Florida, New Jersey, and New York elders and adults with physical disabilities. Submitted for publication to the *Journal of the American Public Health Association*.

Simon-Rusinowitz, L., Bochniak, A. M., Mahoney, K. J., & Hecht, D. (2000). Implementation issues for consumer-directed programs: Views from policy experts. In Kapp, M. B. (Ed.), *Ethics, Law, and Aging Review, Volume 6*. New York: Springer Publishing. 107-129.

Simon-Rusinowitz, L., & Hofland, B. (1993). Adopting a disability approach to home care services for older adults. *The Gerontologist, 33*(2), 159-167.

Simon-Rusinowitz, L., Mahoney, K., Desmond, A., Shoop, D., Squillace, M., & Fay, R. (1997). Determining consumer preferences for a cash option: Arkansas survey results. *Health Care Financing Review 19*(2), 73-96.

Simon-Rusinowitz, L., Mahoney, K. M., Zacharias, B. L., & Marks, L. N. (In Progress). Consumer and representative focus groups inform program design and communication efforts. For submission to *The Gerontologist*.

Stone, R. I. (2000). Consumer direction in long-term care. *Generations, 24*(3), 5-9.

A FEDERAL DEMONSTRATION TO STIMULATE SERVICE DEVELOPMENT WITHIN STATES

Weighing the Success of a National Alzheimer's Disease Service Demonstration

Rhonda J. V. Montgomery, PhD
University of Kansas

Tracy X. Karner, PhD
University of Houston

Karl Kosloski, PhD
University of Nebraska at Omaha

SUMMARY. As the need for long-term care services within the United States has grown dramatically, Congress has consistently deflected the primary responsibility for such care to state governments, local organizations, and, ultimately, the family. This paper examines the impact of the Alzheimer's Disease Demonstration Grants to States (ADDGS) program, a small federally funded initiative within the context of this trend. Although the demonstration can be deemed a huge success relative to the goals of creating new services for an underserved target population,

[Haworth co-indexing entry note]: "Weighing the Success of a National Alzheimer's Disease Service Demonstration." Montgomery, Rhonda J. V., Tracy X. Karner, and Karl Kosloski. Co-published simultaneously in *Journal of Aging & Social Policy* (The Haworth Press, Inc.) Vol. 14, No. 3/4, 2002, pp. 119-139; and: *Devolution and Aging Policy* (ed: Francis G. Caro, and Robert Morris) The Haworth Press, Inc., 2002, pp. 119-139. Single or multiple copies of this article are available for a fee from The Haworth Document Delivery Service [1-800-HAWORTH, 9:00 a.m. - 5:00 p.m. (EST). E-mail address: getinfo@haworthpressinc.com].

10.1300/J031v14n03_07

questions are raised about the merits of the program relative to the exploding need for an effective network of long-term care services. *[Article copies available for a fee from The Haworth Document Delivery Service: 1-800-HAWORTH. E-mail address: <getinfo@haworthpressinc.com> Website: <http://www.HaworthPress.com> © 2002 by The Haworth Press, Inc. All rights reserved.]*

KEYWORDS. Family caregiving, long-term care policy, respite, AoA, Alzheimer's disease, Grants to States Demonstration, National Family Caregiver Support Program, systems development

INTRODUCTION

In the context of the new federalism, which promotes devolution of the responsibility for social problems from the national level to state and local levels, the growing need for long-term care in our society remains a challenge. In the case of care for older adults, this responsibility is deflected *de facto* to the family unit and most often to the unpaid labor of women. The purpose of this paper is to describe a federal demonstration project, the Alzheimer's Disease Demonstration Grant to States (ADDGS), and assess its success within the context of the trend toward devolution. It is argued here that this federal demonstration program, now in its 11th year of operation, serves as a prime example of federal minimalism as a response to a growing and costly societal need.

THE CONTEXT OF LONG-TERM CARE POLICY

The Changing Role of Government

Within the last 25 years, the federal role in domestic health and human services has been restructured through decentralization and devolution movements that have had a great impact on the organization and delivery of long-term care services. Washington has fueled the "devolution revolution" with the increasingly bipartisan conviction that the government closest to the people governs best (Eisinger, 1998). Supporters of devolution have argued that local responsibility will lead to more imaginative and insightful responses to individuals' needs (Borut, 1996), increase consumer choice (Havighurst, 1986), and bring the states into full governing partnerships (Anton, 1997).

Opponents of devolution, however, caution that it will lead to under-funding, inequality, and a "race to the bottom" that will actually dismantle the social safety net (Estes & Linkins, 1997). Furthermore, the use of block grants rather than federal programs allows states greater flexibility to stress universalistic programs rather than particularistic ones that would ensure a certain level of funding for special groups such as the elderly or those in need of long-term care services (Palley, 1997). Finally, devolution practices assume that local governmental units have the resources, infrastructure, and capacity to address social problems and direct programs. Corbett (1997, p. 5) points to a weakness of this assumption, noting, "Flexibility without resources may not be flexibility at all."

A Growing Need for Long-Term Care

While political agendas can be served by the reduction of social programs, "demographic trends signal the urgent need for a long-term care policy solution" (Estes & Linkins, 1997, 428). By 2030, it is projected that one in five U.S. citizens will be over age 65. There also will be large increases in some of the more vulnerable groups, the oldest of the old who live alone, older women, elderly racial minorities living alone, and elderly unmarried persons with no living children and no siblings (Hobbs & Damon, 1996). Moreover, among the fastest-growing segment of America's older population, the oldest old, chronic diseases and disability are most prevalent. In 1990, approximately one quarter of those 85 or older were living in nursing homes, while half of the non-institutionalized among this group required assistance with everyday activities (Hobbs & Damon, 1996). Consequently, as the population continues to age, the demand for long-term care services, including home and community-based assistance, is projected to double or triple (Estes & Linkins, 1997).

Alzheimer's Disease as a Special Case

The need for long-term care is primarily created by physical dependency of elders stemming from a chronic medical condition. Yet, unlike acute medical conditions, there is no entitlement program within the United States to help elders suffering from most chronic conditions to pay for necessary care. This bias in our health care system has frequently been attributed to a bias toward a medical model of care and is particularly problematic for the estimated four million Americans who suffer from Alzheimer's disease. Although Alzheimer's disease is clearly a medical condition, its overt symptoms are primarily behavioral and, currently, incurable. Consequently, the care that is needed by patients with Alzheimer's disease is generally custodial care and not covered by Medicare benefits. Yet, the nature of the disease, which is often associated with problem behaviors, generally places greater demands on both informal and formal care providers.

The deleterious consequences of Alzheimer's disease are not limited to the individuals who are afflicted with the disease, but extend to family members who provide the majority of care for patients (Montgomery & Williams, 2001). To care effectively for persons with Alzheimer's disease, it is important for caregivers to be well versed on behavior management techniques and very familiar with the patient. Although families of Alzheimer's patients are not the only consumers who must cope in the absence of a viable long-term care system, they certainly represent a significant proportion of the population that, daily, encounters the limitations of the system and its providers. In addition to contending with the burdensome costs of care, many families encounter providers of day care, in-home service services, and even residential care that are unwilling or unable to serve clients who are incontinent or who exhibit problem behaviors. Hence, for families dealing with Alzheimer's disease, the situation is grim. Not only is the disease devastating emotionally and physically; it creates a need for a type of care for which there is currently no national system of services.

The Gendered Nature of Our Current Long-Term Care Policies

The need for long-term care is an issue that disproportionately impacts women because the majority of older Americans are women and the majority of family caregivers are women. Long-term care policy generally has emphasized the benefits of community-based care over formal, institutional care, and has been accompanied by a greater expectation for family care. This expectation for relatives to provide direct care remains more implicit than explicit in written policies (Doty, 1995). For example, changes in Medicare coverage related to the prospective payment system have resulted in shorter hospital stays for elders who are now being discharged with greater needs for assistance (Estes & Swan, 1993). The assumption appears to be that family members are, or should be, available to provide the needed care (Montgomery, 1999). This deflection of responsibility for long-term care to families also is evident in screening processes mandated by many states for elders seeking admission into nursing homes and in the eligibility requirements for Supplemental Security Income (SSI), which reduce benefits for individuals who live with other persons or who receive in-kind contributions from others (Hendricks & Hatch, 1993). It is within this context of the growing national need for long-term care, federal minimalism, and the deflection of responsibility for this care to families that the Alzheimer's Disease Demonstration Grants to States (ADDGS) program emerged and its relative success must be assessed.

DESCRIPTION OF THE ALZHEIMER'S DISEASE DEMONSTRATION GRANTS TO STATES PROGRAM

Enabling Legislation

In response to advocacy efforts, legislation was passed in 1990 for a small service demonstration, which was placed in the U.S. Department of Health and Human Services Bureau of Primary Care of the Health Resources Services Administration (HRSA). The Alzheimer's Disease Demonstration Grant to States Program (ADDGS) was authorized through Sections 398, 399, and 399A of the Public Health Service (PHS) Act, as amended by Public Law 101-557 Home Health Care and Alzheimer's Disease Amendments of 1990. The demonstration program was intended to assist grantees in planning, establishing, and operating demonstration programs in the following areas:

1. program development,
2. services delivery, and
3. information dissemination.

The legislation was particularly intended to help states deliver support services to hard-to-serve and underserved populations, which were generally defined as rural and ethnic minority populations.

The demonstration was initially authorized for three years with funding of three million dollars. Since that time, the legislation has been reauthorized three times, extending the demonstration through 2005 and increasing its annual funding to almost eleven million dollars. In 1998, in keeping with its primary mission to serve elderly clients, the demonstration was moved administratively within the Department of Health and Human Services from HRSA to the Administration on Aging (AoA).

The focus of this article is on the demonstration projects undertaken by the initial 15 grantees. Grantees were selected through two rounds of competitive requests for proposals. In September of 1992, nine states (California, Florida, Maine, Maryland, Michigan, Montana, Ohio, Oregon, South Carolina), Puerto Rico, and the District of Columbia were selected to receive a three-year demonstration grant. In July of 1993, four additional states received a demonstration grant (Georgia, Hawaii, North Carolina, Washington).

Evaluation Activities

In compliance with the enabling legislation, an evaluation has been conducted throughout the implementation process. Initially, the evaluation design included both a descriptive component and an outcome component focused on three broad sets of questions:

1. What services were developed and how were they delivered?
2. Who was served and how satisfied were they?
3. What strategies did grantees use that facilitated the development and delivery of support services?

In late 1996, the evaluation activities shifted to a limited description of client intakes and the monthly use of direct care services. Finally, in 1999, the AoA extended evaluation activities to include analysis of longitudinal data related to patterns of respite use, and a survey of elder services clients and staff focused on cultural issues related to service delivery and use. The central focus of this endeavor was to understand better:

1. how families use respite services,
2. how families evaluate respite services in light of their beliefs, culture, and need, and
3. how providers can develop appropriate and successful respite services.

Evaluation data were gathered from seven sources: client records, program/employee records, client satisfaction interviews, site visits, review of project documents, telephone consultations and an intensive two-day workshop with key informants.[1] Data pertaining to clients were collected at the time of initial contact and at the time of enrollment for services. Additionally, records were maintained documenting the date and amount of each incident of service delivery for each client. Data pertaining to client satisfaction were gathered through interviews conducted with 1,311 primary caregivers, including 222 family members who contacted the program, but did not receive services. Details relating to the sampling design are reported in Montgomery et al., 1997.

Data describing program development and service characteristics were reported by project personnel using standard data collection forms pertaining to employee characteristics, outreach, education and training, activities, and service descriptions. Additionally, in-depth information about program development and challenges to implementation was obtained through site visits and reviews of initial proposals, quarterly reports, and annual reports prepared by each grantee. Telephone interviews were conducted with key representatives of each grantee at several points throughout the demonstration to clarify information and obtain additional information when necessary. (See Montgomery et al., 1997 and 2002 for a full discussion.) Finally, in June 1997, a small two-day workshop was conducted with nine key informants who represented eight of the grantee programs. This workshop consisted of a series of focus groups and in-person interviews intended to identify and explore, in depth, issues and barriers related to successful development of programs that were likely to continue beyond the demonstration and serve as models for replication. (See Service Models at *http:// www.aoa.gov/alz/brochures.*) Together, these multiple sources provide a rich database that can be used to explore the success of the demonstration.

Unique and Guiding Characteristics of the Demonstration

To describe and understand ADDGS within the context of devolution, it is useful to identify several characteristics of the demonstration that have influenced its implementation and, ultimately, its success in meeting the goals of multiple stakeholders. First, the demonstration was characterized by great flexibility. Unlike many demonstrations linked to entitlement programs, the ADDGS allowed grantees considerable latitude for designing local programs and use of funds. The only restriction placed on use of funds was the requirement that 50% of the funds be used for respite services.[2] Furthermore, each of the states was given latitude in designating the state agency that would receive the funds and serve as the lead agency. States were encouraged to work with and through agencies outside of the traditional network of aging services, and most did.

A second requirement of the demonstration was the inclusion in the project of an organization with expertise about Alzheimer's disease and experience working in some capacity with families affected by the disease. Most often this meant the inclusion of a local chapter of the Alzheimer's Association. Consequently, it also meant the formation of partnerships between public and private organizations in every demonstration site.

A corollary of the flexibility that characterized the demonstration was the expectation at the federal level for innovation and experimentation, which was accompanied by a tolerance for initial failures. For example, when the project in Georgia encountered numerous obstacles to replicating in rural settings a community-based program first implemented in an urban community, the state was able to shift funds to new programs that were successful in later years.

A third defining characteristic of the demonstration was the intent of the legislation to support a very small and circumscribed program. The demonstration was not focused on the broad group of families facing long-term care needs for elderly members. Instead, it was narrowly focused on a small group of hard-to-reach families confronting the challenges of Alzheimer's disease. Hence, it could not be construed as a long-term care program that had any likelihood of being expanded to an entitlement program. Moreover, the requirement for matching funds from the grantees increased from 25% in the first year to 45% by the third year, all but ensuring state governments and local organizations share responsibility for the continuance of service programs.

Stakeholders and Their Goals

Although the stated goal for each of the grantees and their participating partner organizations was the creation of new support services for hard-to-reach families caring for persons with Alzheimer's disease, the demonstration provided an opportunity for at least four sets of stakeholders simultaneously to address differing long-term or short-term goals. At the federal level, the program was aimed at serving segments of the elderly population that had considerable unmet needs for long-term care. A second, but unstated, goal was to serve this population in a manner that would not create a new entitlement program or entrench the program in an ongoing bureaucratic structure. The temporary nature of the program was essentially ensured by both the demonstration status of the program and its limited funding, which precluded development of any program fully meeting the needs of even this very select population, much less the long-term care needs of the general elderly population. In short, the demonstration served as a small catalyst program to facilitate the deflection of responsibility for long-term care from the federal level to the state level and, ultimately, to the family. The goal was to help families assume responsibility for meeting the needs. While recognizing the needs of families confronting long-term care, the program simultaneously avoided any imagery that might convey an assumption of responsibility for long-term care by the federal government.

State governments were the second set of stakeholders participating in the demonstration, with a state agency designated as the lead grantee. In thirteen states, grants were awarded to the state unit on aging. The state agency for mental health served as a lead agency in Michigan and as a key partner in the states of South Carolina and California. The state department of health served as the grantee in California. From the perspective of state governments, the demonstration was an opportunity to procure a new stream of federal funds for long-term care services. Through collaborative efforts, state agencies were able to propose and implement the extension of existing programs or the creation of new programs by obtaining new funds. Like the federal government, however, many of the state agencies treated the demonstration as a temporary resource that would facilitate the shifting of long-term care costs to local communities or the retention of costs by family members. In some cases, the demonstration funds were used to support existing programs, replacing state funds that were then shifted to other uses.

The third set of stakeholders, local community organizations, was the most diverse. As indicated in Table 1, there was wide variation across the fifteen grantees in the numbers and types of local organizations that participated. This third set of stakeholders included local social service agencies, home health agencies, chapters of the Alzheimer's Association, local health departments, and community health and social services owned and operated by ethnic minority groups. Like the state agencies, many of the local organizations participating in the ADDGS viewed the demonstration funds as a new resource that could be used to extend ongoing but financially tenuous programs or to support new programs. For example, several of the local chapters of the Alzheimer's Association were able to use the demonstration funds to create a stable staff that could then extend outreach and direct services to the general population of Alzheimer's families as well as to the targeted populations. Other local programs were able to use the federal dollars as seed funds to entice local agencies to create Alzheimer's-friendly services and to extend existing services to the target populations.

The fourth group of stakeholders consisted of the client families who were directly served by the demonstration programs. When faced with the option of retaining complete responsibility for long-term care or receiving some help with this responsibility, this client group was unlikely to voice opposition to any program that offered even a small window of relief. Few, if any, of the clients focused their attention on the more basic issue or question of ultimate responsibility for long-term care. For the most part, this client population could be characterized as having limited political voice as well as limited awareness of the implications of the ADDGS in terms of delegation of responsibility for long-term care.

Services Developed and Delivered

As noted above, the ADDGS has been characterized by considerable local diversity in design and implementation. While every grantee was responsible for the creation of respite services and outreach for hard-to-reach populations, each state (and territory) was encouraged to develop and implement a program of outreach and support services specific to its unique needs and resources. Every grantee state developed three types of services: outreach and education opportunities, respite services, and other direct services intended to support families. The exact form and quantity of these common services, however, varied widely across the fifteen grantees. (Full descriptions of the services offered through the demonstration may be found in Montgomery et al., 1997.)

During the first four years of operation, 6,938 clients were enrolled in the demonstration, and received 1,039,506 units of respite and direct support services. In-home respite (515,872 hours) and adult day care (451,904 hours) were the most prevalent services utilized. By the end of the ninth year of the demonstration, the fifteen grantees had directly served 14,407 clients providing over 3,500,000 units of service and successfully reaching the targeted underserved and hard-to-reach populations. Regardless of geographic location, fully half of the participants were ethnic minorities with 19.4% being African American, 22.5% Hispanic, 6.8% Asian or Pacific Islander, and 1% Native American. Half of the participants for whom geographic location was recorded (53% or 44.9% of the total sample) resided in rural areas (Montgomery et al., 2002).

ASSESSING THE SUCCESS OF THE DEMONSTRATION

Success as Service Delivery

Given the multiple stakeholders and multiple goals of the ADDGS, success may be defined and measured in a number of ways. At the most basic level, the demonstration could be declared successful to the extent

TABLE 1. Key Characterstics of Grantee Programs

State	Target Population	Number of Sites*	Key Partners	Type(s) of Respite	Other Support Services**	Primary Initiative(s)	Families Served
California	Hispanic/Latino	3 urban	State Depts. of Health Services, Aging, Mental Health and Social Services AA-Chapters Local Service Delivery Local Minority Service Delivery	ADC Social day In-home Institutional	Legal assistance Support groups Translation	Hispanic/Latino communities	267
District of Columbia	African American	4 urban	DC Office on Aging AA-Chapters Local Service Delivery	ADC In-home Residental	Support groups	Elders living alone	309
Florida	Hispanic Cuban American African American Rural	6 urban 1 rural	State Dept. of Elder Affairs AA-Chapters Local Service Delivery Local Minority Service Delivery	ADC In-home (vol.) In-home (paid) Institutional	Diagnosis Support groups	Volunteer-based respite	787
Georgia	African American Rural	7 rural	State Dept. of Aging Services AAAs AA-Chapters Local Service Delivery	ADC Social day In-home Institutional	Home safety Chores	Mobile day care Assistive technology Home modification	94
Hawaii	Filipino Native Hawaiian Vietnamese	12 urban	State Dept. of Aging AA-Chapters Local Minority Service Delivery	In-home (vol.) In-home (paid) ADC		Asian/Pacific Islander communities	268
Maine	Franco Americans Rural	4 rural	State Dept. of Elder & Adult Services AAAs AA-Chapters Local Service Delivery	In-home (vol.) In-home (paid) Social day Residential	Diagnosis and assessment Counseling	Dementia assessment teams for rural elders	308
Maryland	African American Rural	1 urban 3 rural	State Dept. of Adult Services AA-Chapters Local Service Delivery	In-home ADC Residential	Support groups	Respite voucher program	504
Michigan	African American Rural	1 urban 20 rural	State Dept. of Community Health AA-Chapters AAAs Local Service Delivery Local Health Delivery	In-home (vol.) In-home (paid) ADC	Diagnosis Support group Counseling	African-American and rural communities	390
Montana	Native American Rural	3 rural	State Dept. of Senior & Long Term Care State Dept. of Aging AAAs AA-Chapters Local Minority Health Delivery	In-home		Native American communities	47

TABLE 1 (continued)

State	Target Population	Number of Sites*	Key Partners	Type(s) of Respite	Other Support Services**	Primary Initiative(s)	Families Served
North Carolina	African American Rural	14 rural	State Dept. of Aging AA-Chapters Local Service Delivery Local Health Delivery	In-home ADC Social day		Social day care for African American and rural communities	142
Ohio	Rural	4 urban	State Dept. of Aging AA-Chapters		800 Helpline	Family directed care management	292
Oregon	Rural	4 urban 10 rural	State Dept.of Senior & Disabled Services AA-Chapters AAAs Local Service Delivery Local Health Delivery	Social day	Support groups	Case mgmt training Brookdale models	167
Puerto Rico	Puerto Ricans Rural	4 urban 4 rural	Dept. of Elder Affairs AAAs Local Health Delivery	In-home	Diagnosis Support group Counseling	Puerto Rican community	289
South Carolina	Rural	3 urban 10 rural	State Depts. of Aging, Mental Health AAAs AA-Chapters Local Service Delivery Local Health Delivery	In-home ADC Institutional		African American and rural communities	279
Washington	Chinese Korean Hispanic Native American Rural	3 urban 1 rural	State Dept. of Aging and Adult Services AAAs Local Service Delivery Local Health Delivery	In-home ADC Residential	Support groups Translation	Dementia education Client advocacy	236

*Communities in which respite programs were implemented, in many cases multiple agencies provided support services in these communities.
**In addition to respite and case management.

130

that new support services were created and delivered to the targeted populations. Equally important to the goals of the federal and state governments, there is much evidence that the demonstration successfully served as a catalyst to promote development of a wide range of new, locally based programs that offer support services.

Success as Program Stability

Many of the local organizations participating in the ADDGS were able to use the demonstration funds as a new resource to extend ongoing programs that were financially tenuous or to support new programs. New support programs implemented in these communities were still in operation at the end of a 9-year funding period and are likely to continue beyond the duration of the demonstration. However, this outcome was not uniform. To gain insight into activities contributing to the long-term stability of demonstration projects, available data were examined.

Just as there was great variation among the programs in the services developed, there also was great diversity in the infrastructure and resources available to the grantees as well as in the processes they used to develop services. Scrutiny of project reports, site visits, interviews with key personnel, and the focused meeting with key personnel revealed community commitment and creation of new resources as two elements that were common to the most successful demonstrations. Community commitment and the creation of new resources appeared to be requisites for the creation of programs that had the potential to endure beyond the demonstration period.

Building Community Commitment as a Requisite for Success

Program administrators repeatedly noted that successful development and delivery of support services hinged upon involvement of local agencies and organizations and their commitment to the new program. Administrators in several states identified the importance of a broad based coalition of community agencies to the success of local programs. Staff of successful programs cautioned against placing all local resources into one agency and expressed the belief that state agencies should require, as a condition of funding, evidence of local interagency commitment to collaborate and improve coordination. This advice was given with the recognition that individual agencies in economically depressed communities may not be able to provide the required 25% local match. A single agency also may not have the needed leadership skills in program and community development.

Forging of New Partnerships. The necessary level of community ownership and collaboration frequently required the development of new or stronger links between organizations and service systems that had been operating independently of one another. Strong partnerships were especially critical for the development of new or previously unserved or underserved populations. These newly created partnerships promoted collaboration that led to better coordination of service delivery among service organizations, significant improvement in service infrastructures, and, ultimately, a greater capacity to serve ethnically diverse populations.

Expanding Awareness. To gain the commitment of local communities to the demonstration programs, it was important for the programs' staff to expand the awareness of community members about both the prevalence of Alzheimer's disease and the needs of caregivers. This increased awareness is a prominent legacy of the national demonstration. Its impact has been especially beneficial in rural areas and among ethnic communities.

The expansion of awareness has been an iterative process working in tandem with partnership development. To promote strong organizational partnerships, each partner had to be informed of the needs of elders and families in their respective constituencies. At the same time, strong partnerships served as a foundation for increasing awareness within the community at large of the needs of families and of service availability. These initial outreach efforts to public and private partnerships created links to the community. Foundational support was rallied through the involvement of local individuals in the planning processes. For example, in California the formation of community advisory councils, a steering committee, a community task group, and a multidisciplinary demonstration team have broadened the support network of the demonstration project within the Latino community. This, in turn, served both to promote the project and to develop linkages among existing agencies and providers.[3]

Generally, the process of building strong partnerships generated trust and support from respected members of the community, and this trust was essential for generating acceptance of new services within minority ethnic communities. The simple availability and awareness of respite care services does not necessarily result in the use of such services. Project staff found that successful promotion of the program requires both time and effort contacting and partnering with key community leaders and ethnic physicians.

In the states of Michigan and California, the demonstration served as an impetus to create or improve coordination between the state units on aging and departments of health or mental health-related units at the state level. Similarly, at the local level, new partnerships and collaborations among the aging networks, local health departments, and community health providers have resulted from the demonstrations in the states of Maryland, North Carolina, Oregon, South Carolina, and Washington. The fruitful relationship of medical and social agencies has benefited each agency's reputation and credibility.

Generation of New Resources Essential to Success

Through strong partnerships that generated community commitment, many demonstration programs were able to create and acquire resources essential to building the capacity of communities to serve Alzheimer families. Technical support in the form of expertise for training and education efforts was critical for building the capacity of staff to serve persons with Alzheimer's disease. Additionally, new funding sources were necessary to expand existing services and support new programs beyond the period of demonstration funds.

Importance of Adequate Technical Support to Success. Ongoing technical support for outreach, training, and educational efforts was particularly useful to demonstration projects located in remote rural areas, which tend to be isolated from educational opportunities and resources. New service programs benefited significantly from training programs for their own staff and for staff of service partners. Technical support to local demonstration projects in the form of professional expertise also enriched outreach programs directed toward the general community and educational programs for family members.

Staff members from the North Carolina sites deemed technical support critical to the success of their outreach, training, and education efforts, which, to cultivate development and use of services in hard-to-reach communities, was a continual processes. In all of the North Carolina sites, staff indicated that their initial expectations regarding the need for education about Alzheimer's disease and the benefits of support services had been significantly underestimated. Staff in Oregon, Michigan, Maine, Washington, Puerto Rico, and South Carolina echoed these sentiments.

New Funding as a Means to Stability. One of the primary goals of the demonstration was to facilitate the development of programs that would continue beyond the demonstration period. The continuation of services has been fostered in two ways. In some states, demonstration services have been integrated into existing service systems and continue to operate under existing state or local programs. This mechanism has been used in North Carolina to continue respite care, in Oregon to continue training of case managers, and in Florida to continue the group respite programs. In other states, the coalitions of service agencies that emerged through the ADDGS demonstration have worked to locate and develop new resources to support continuance of demonstration services. In several cases, collaboration between the local Alzheimer's Association chapters and community service providers has created strong advocacy groups for resource development. In other cases, strong partners have collaborated to apply for additional public and private funds to develop new services or to support the demonstration services in the future. Particularly successful resource development has taken place in Michigan, South Carolina, and California.[4]

Success as Deflection of Responsibility

Although there was wide variation across the fifteen grantees in stability and longevity of programs, the final reports of most of the grantees indicate that at least some portion of state or local support services initiated under the auspices of the demonstration was expected to continue to operate after the demonstration funds ended. Furthermore, in several sites the growth of the initial project programs has been fostered through the use of local resources, and the projects have provided a foundation for more widely based growth in respite services across the states. Two examples of such growth can be found in Maine and California.

In the case of Maine, the demonstration successfully served as a catalyst for generating a commitment of state dollars to support programs that help families to continue as primary sources of long-term care. Resource development efforts of the Maine program resulted in the state legislature allocating over nine million dollars to develop and implement a community-based system. Within the context of the federal agenda for minimalism, this expansion of dollars at the state level for respite services might well be considered a success.

In the case of California, the deflection of responsibility for long-term care has proceeded a step beyond the state. The California project serves as an example of a local community taking on the responsibility for long-term care services and generating the necessary resources to support the care program. Again, however, the newly implemented long-term care services are focused on maintaining the family as the primary source of long-term care with support being provided to the family.

The original goal of the California project known as El Portal was to develop and provide culturally and linguistically competent educational, medical, social, and supportive services for Hispanic/Latino dementia-affected persons, their families, and caregivers. At the time that ADDGS funds were granted to the state of California, about 36% of the nine million persons residing in Los Angeles County were Latino or Hispanic. Yet there were no dementia-specific services targeting Latinos in the geographic area.

Through a unique collaborative effort involving government, consumers, providers, academia, and the communities, El Portal developed a network of services that has been fostered by the ADDGS (*http://www.aoa.gov/alz/brochures*). At the midpoint in the grant-funding period, El Portal partner agencies formed a work group to collaborate on strategies to maintain the program after the Alzheimer's Demonstration funds ended. Collaborative grant writing and funding requests generated over $800,000 by the end of the fifth year of operation and other initiatives were pending at that time. Additionally, the initial demonstration site was positioned to receive state funds through the California Department of Aging.

These examples of mobilization of local resources point to the success of ADDGS with helping to deflect the responsibility for long-term care responsibilities from the states to local entities. The ADDGS has provided funds necessary to support processes of development in local communities that can be costly in dollars and time and often do not immediately produce direct services for client families.

Viewing Success as Setting a Precedent

While proponents of federal minimalism might point to the deflection of responsibility for long-term care programs to state and local entities as a marker of success, opponents of such minimalism might take heart in the precedent that the ADDGS has set for a federal presence in the creation of long-term care services. The success of the program in fostering services for Alzheimer's families has not gone unrecognized by Congress. Rather, the enabling legislation has been reauthorized three times, and the annual budget has been tripled. Moreover, 25 states have received new grants in the past year and there are currently congressional bills in progress that are seeking the expansion of the program. All of this portends a steady progression of growth in long-term care services under the auspices of the federal government.

Additionally, the ADDGS has served as a source of critical information to guide the implementation of the newly created AoA National Family Caregiver Support Program (see *www.aoa.gov*). As the Administration on Aging has moved forward with the implementation of its first new major initiative in 20 years, key staff members have looked to administrators and providers of programs funded through the ADDGS for insights. Additionally, findings from the ongoing evaluation have provided critical information that has been shared with program administrators and providers throughout the country through online listservs and national and local workshops. In all of these ways, the ADDGS might be seen as successful in promoting the presence of the federal government in the delivery of long-term care services.

Success of the Demonstration as an Influence on Long-Term Care Policy

While the ADDGS can be judged hugely successful in some ways, it might also be considered problematic when evaluated in a broader context. Against the criteria of promoting fairness and adequacy of long-term care policy, the ADDGS might be viewed as not addressing three specific needs. First as a demonstration, the program was limited in scope by its focus on a select target population. Targeted only to clients with Alzheimer's disease in 15 states, the demonstration did not address needs of the full range of older adults and their families who confront the challenges of long-term care. Instead, it was focused on a limited group of rural and minority populations.

Second, the demonstration did not result in an equitable distribution of federal resources to needy families and communities. Initially, the different states were at different levels of readiness to compete for and implement the demonstration. Thus, award levels varied by grantee. Moreover, evidence from the evaluation suggests that states with stronger infrastructures, greater resources, and more highly skilled staff were better able to use the federal dollars to build service systems that had the greatest potential to endure beyond the demonstration. The states and communities that initially had the weakest infrastructures and fewest initial resources also encountered the greatest challenges to effective implementation of programs with any likelihood of endurance. Consequently, the support programs in these sites, which included Puerto Rico, Montana, the Korean and Native American Communities in Washington, and some rural communities in Oregon, South Carolina, North Carolina, and Michigan, did not continue beyond the end of the demonstration.

Most problematic is the possibility that the ADDGS will divert the attention of Congress from the larger need for a national system for delivery of long-term care services that does not rest on the assumption that the family is, and will continue to be, available to provide care for older adults. The fact that long-term care continues to be a complex and growing problem that will be costly and difficult to address does not excuse our reluctance as a society to acknowledge our responsibility to care for the vulnerable and needy among us.

If the ADDGS serves to reinforce the notion that long-term care needs are family responsibilities, then it reinforces the belief that these needs are private troubles, rather than social problems to be addressed through federal policy. Translated into practice, this philosophy means that families must continue to assume the ultimate responsibility for long-term care and that unpaid or low-paid women will provide the majority of care. Consequently, the philosophy serves as a strong reinforcement of stereotypic gender norms and of repressive policy that is blind to the inequities of a health care system that ignores the needs of individuals who suffer from chronic disabilities and their families.

CONCLUSION

The final verdict regarding the success of the ADDGS will depend on how information gained from the demonstration is used to guide policy and practice in the future. If, in the end, the ADDGS turns out to have been a small, focused response that deflected attention away from the larger national need for equitable access to long-term care, the program will not have achieved its full potential for success. On the other hand, if, in addition to supporting programs to meet the pressing long-term care needs within states and local communities, the demonstration serves as a source of valuable information that can guide policy makers to a fuller consideration of the potential inequities associated with the current medical model of long-term care, its impact may be extremely positive.

NOTES

1. A full description of the data collection forms and the forms themselves are included in the final report: Montgomery et al. (1997). *Alzheimer's Demonstration Grant to States, 1992-1996. Final Evaluation Report to the Health Resources Services Administration.* January.

2. This requirement and other requirements for matched funds were included in the requests for proposals issued by HRSA and AoA.

3. A detailed description of the California El Portal project can be found at: *http://www.aoa.gov/alz/brochures/brochures_main.asp.*

4. More detailed descriptions of the resource development efforts can be found in: Montgomery et al. (1997). *Alzheimer's Demonstration Grant to States, 1992-1996. Final Evaluation Report to the Health Resources Services Administration.* January.

AUTHOR NOTES

Rhonda J. V. Montgomery is Director of the Gerontology Center at the University of Kansas and Professor of Sociology. She is the principal investigator for the Administration on Aging National Alzheimer's Disease Grants to States demonstration program. Her research interests focus on the role of the family in long-term care.

Dr. Montgomery can be contacted at the Gerontology Center-University of Kansas, Dole Human Development Center, 1000 Sunnyside Ave., Room 3090, Lawrence, KS 66045-7555 (E-mail: rmontgomery@ukans.edu).

Tracy X. Karner is Assistant Professor of Sociology at the University of Houston. She served as Project Director for the ADDGS evaluation during the first wave of grantees. Dr. Karner's research interests include medical sociology, gender, and social change.

Dr. Karner can be contacted at the Department of Sociology, University of Houston, 450 Philip Hoffman Hall, Houston, TX 77204.

Karl Kosloski is Professor of Gerontology and Reynolds Professor of Public Policy at the University of Nebraska at Omaha. His research interests include retirement planning, the use of supportive services by informal caregivers of Alzheimer's patients, caregiving outcomes, measurement issues, and program evaluation.

Dr. Kosloski can be contacted at the University of Nebraska at Omaha, Department of Gerontology, 6001 Dodge St., Omaha, NE 68182.

REFERENCES

Anton, T. J. (1997). New federalism and intergovernmental fiscal relationships: The implications for health policy. *Journal of Health Politics, Policy, and Law, 22*(3), 691-720.

Borut, D. (1996). Aspirations and accountability: Local government in the era of devolution. *National Civic Review, 85,* 23-27.

Corbett, T. (1997). *Informing the welfare debate: Perspectives on the transformation of social policy.* Institute for Research on Poverty, Special Report no. 70.

Doty, P. (1995). Family caregiving and access to publicly funded home care. In R. A. Kane & J. D. Penrod (Eds.), *Family caregiving in an aging society* (pp. 92-122). Thousand Oaks, CA: Sage Publications, Inc.

Eisinger, P. (1998). City politics in an era of federal devolution. *Urban Affairs Review, 33*(3), 308-325.

Estes, C. L., & Linkins, K. W. (1997). Devolution and aging policy: Racing to the bottom in long-term care. *International Journal of Health Services, 27*(3), 427-442.

Estes, C. L., & Swan, J. H. (1993). *The long-term care crisis.* Newbury Park, CA: Sage Publications, Inc.

Havighurst, C. C. (1986) The changing locus of decision making in the health care sector. *Journal of Health Politics, Policy, and Law, 11*(4), 697-735.

Hendricks, J., & Hatch, L. R. (1993). Federal policy and family life of older Americans. In J. Hendricks & C. J. Rosenthal (Eds.), *The remainder of their days: Domestic policy and older families in the United States and Canada* (pp. 49-73). New York: Garland Publishing, Inc.

Hobbs, F. B., & Damon, B. L. (1996). *65+ in the United States.* U.S. Census: Current Population Reports, Special Studies.

Montgomery, R. J. V. (1999). The family role in the context of long-term care. *Journal of Aging and Health, 11*(3), 401-434.

Montgomery, R. J. V. (Ed.) (2002). A new look at respite programs: Utilization, satisfaction & development. *Home Health Care Quarterly* (Special Issue), *21*(3/4).

Montgomery, R. J. V., Karner, T. X., Kosloski, K. D. Schaefer, J. P., Hupp, K., Klaus, S., & Schleyer, M. (2001). *Further analysis and evaluation of the Administration on Aging Alzheimer's Disease Demonstration Grant to States.* Report to the Administration on Aging. Lawrence, KS.

Montgomery, R. J. V., Kosloski, K. D., Karner, T. X., Hall, L. C., & Schaefer, J. P. (1997). *Alzheimer's demonstration grant to states project: Final evaluation report to Bureau of Primary Health Care.* Health Resources Services Administration. Lawrence, KS.

Montgomery, R. J. V., Kosloski, K. D., Karner, T. X., & Schaefer, J. P. (2002). The Alzheimer's Disease Demonstration Grant to States Program. *Home Health Care Quarterly* (Special Issue), *21*(3/4).

Montgomery, R. J. V., & Williams, K. (2001). Implications of differential impacts of caregiving for the future research on Alzheimer care. *The Journal of Aging and Mental Health,* May 5 (Supplement 1), S23-S34.

Palley, M. L. (1997). Intergovernmentalization of health care reform: The limits of the devolution revolution. *Journal of Politics, 59*(3), 657-679.

PUBLIC SECTOR, STATE, AND LOCAL INITIATIVES

Strengthening Senior Tax Credit Programs in Massachusetts

Kristin Kiesel, MA

University of Massachusetts Boston

SUMMARY. In the last decade, property taxes have increased, creating a financial burden on senior homeowners. In Massachusetts, senior property tax credit programs have arisen to address this problem, as well as to provide cost-effective volunteer assistance for municipal departments, offer seniors meaningful work that otherwise would not have been attempted, and foster involvement in municipal government among seniors. The success of the programs in retaining senior homeowners in the community remains to be evaluated. Program specifics are detailed, policy options are considered, and recommendations are made to strengthen existing programs and assist replication. *[Article copies available for a fee from The Haworth Document Delivery Service: 1-800-HAWORTH. E-mail address: <getinfo@haworthpressinc.com> Website: <http://www.HaworthPress.com> © 2002 by The Haworth Press, Inc. All rights reserved.]*

[Haworth co-indexing entry note]: "Strengthening Senior Tax Credit Programs in Massachusetts." Kiesel, Kristin. Co-published simultaneously in *Journal of Aging & Social Policy* (The Haworth Press, Inc.) Vol. 14, No. 3/4, 2002, pp. 141-159; and: *Devolution and Aging Policy* (ed: Francis G. Caro, and Robert Morris) The Haworth Press, Inc., 2002, pp. 141-159. Single or multiple copies of this article are available for a fee from The Haworth Document Delivery Service [1-800-HAWORTH, 9:00 a.m. - 5:00 p.m. (EST). E-mail address: getinfo@haworthpressinc.com].

10.1300/J031v14n03_08

KEYWORDS. Senior volunteers, tax credit, government volunteers, productive aging, senior tax policy

INTRODUCTION

Older adults across Massachusetts have faced a taxing dilemma in recent years. As property taxes have risen, those on fixed incomes become less able to afford to remain homeowners in communities where, in many cases, they have spent most of their adult lives.

Several communities in Massachusetts have attempted to promote community service while reducing the impact of property taxes for people on fixed incomes by offering versions of a "tax work-off" plan. The chief provision of the plan is that participants (usually elders) agree to perform a particular number of hours of work for their municipality in return for a property tax credit. The first such plan was introduced in 1992 in Chelmsford, a town of 34,000 north of Boston. It emerged at the grassroots level, promoted by the Council on Aging as a means of assisting senior residents of the town with an average annual property tax bill of $3,400. The program spread rapidly and informally from one municipality to another in eastern Massachusetts. Currently, more than 50 cities and towns have adopted versions of the plan.

The goals of these plans are similar. They include the retention of seniors in the community by reducing their tax burdens, the provision of qualified workers for municipal departments and functions at a low cost to the municipality, the ability to accomplish meaningful work that otherwise would not have been attempted, and an increase of interest and involvement in municipal government and affairs among seniors.

PROBLEM ANALYSIS

People reach retirement age with varying assets in both income and possessions. Many elder homeowners, especially those who have reached age 70 and beyond, find themselves in an unenviable position.

As they have lived in their homes, the value of their property has tended to increase due to the growing demand for housing and the limited amount of land available for home construction, especially in areas close to urban centers where most jobs are located. For many elders, the mortgage has long since been repaid, but property taxes have risen steeply enough that they greatly outweigh any putative savings from the absence of a monthly mortgage payment.

At the same time, many elders are living on fixed incomes. Even though Social Security payments increase annually in an attempt to match the rising cost of living, the increased expense for Medicare Part B (deducted from the monthly Social Security check) has also risen. Elders who worked may have private pensions, but most of these pensions yield a fixed payment, the value of which decreases annually with inflation. Eventually, savings and investments must be tapped in order to continue to pay property taxes.

The length of time people spend in retirement has expanded, and time that was formerly used for work is often used for passive activities like watching television (Fischer & Schaeffer, 1993, p. 7). Retired people not only lose the role identity that being employed gave them; they also lose their sense of being of value, sometimes to the extent that they no longer believe life is worth living (Herzog & House, 1991). Volunteering can provide an antidote for the feeling of valuelessness, especially when it couples meaningful activity with demonstrated benefit for both the volunteer and the organization (Brudney, 1990).

Brudney's research indicates that when municipalities feel under financial stress, they establish mechanisms that encourage greater voluntary involvement among residents (Brudney, 1990, 13), but when the first tax work-off programs were adopted, many Massachusetts cities and towns were financially secure. The range of options available to seniors seeking property tax relief included state property tax exemption and deferral programs such as Clause 17D, a $175 exemption for people age 70 and older who had owned and occupied their home for at least five years, and whose estate was not worth more than $40,000; Clause 18, which allows municipal Boards of Assessors to exempt a portion of the tax for people who, because of age, infirmities, or financial conditions, are unable to pay; Clause 22, providing a $175 exemption for certain veterans and their spouses; Clause 37A, providing a $437.50 exemption for blind homeowners; Clause 41A, which allows property holders with annual incomes of $40,000 or less to defer property taxes under certain circumstances (the deferred taxes become a lien on the property that must be paid when the estate is settled); and Clause 41C, which allows a $500 abatement for people age 70 and older with very low income and assets. Except for benefits for disabled veterans, only one of these options is allowed per household each year. Each of these programs is applicable only to limited groups of residents, and many are not attractive to residents because they appear to be a form of charity.

The tax work-off programs, on the other hand, had the advantage of allowing seniors to trade valuable services for their tax benefits.

Seniors may also take advantage of "Reverse Mortgage" plans, under which a lending institution provides regular cash payments or a lump sum against the value of the property. Borrowers must be at least 62 years of age and occupy the home as their principal residence. The current maximum reverse mortgage in Massachusetts is $262,000. Enrolling in the reverse mortgage program does not exempt property owners from property taxes (AARP, 2002). Many seniors are resistant to taking advantage of this plan. They are averse to increasing their debt burden at a time when their income may be needed for medical expenses, and are aware that should the full value of their homes be "borrowed" under a reverse mortgage, they might be forced to sell their homes in order to repay the loan. In addition, the equity value in their home decreases, and little may be left for heirs.

Volunteering is prompted by a variety of motives, including an impetus to fill the vocational void left by retirement, to continue to feel useful by helping others (Barlow & Hainsworth, 2001), for the opportunity to have social contact with others (Wilson & Musik, 1999), and for various personal and ideological reasons (Fischer & Schaeffer, 1993). People likely to volunteer have more years of education, feel themselves to be in good health, and may have higher incomes than those less likely to volunteer (Cheang, Braun, & Sheeran, 2001). The property tax work-off programs were developed to address the problem of rising taxes and to take advantage of the available skills of senior residents, without regard to socioeconomic status.

METHODS

Telephone and/or in-person interviews were conducted with a snowball sample of respondents, beginning with a list of participating municipalities obtained from the Massachusetts Executive Office of Elder Affairs. The interviewees included Directors of Councils on Aging (10), elected officials (2), department heads (2), the Executive Director of the Massachusetts Service Alliance, and tax work-off participants (2) using a structured interview guide and open-ended questions. Additional information was gathered from newspaper reports and from documents provided by Council on Aging staff, including written testimonials from department heads and completed satisfaction surveys from participants.

Virtually no empirical data are yet available, and the programs are inconsistent with regard to tracking of demographic information on participation. The grassroots nature of the movement as it has arisen over the last decade has resulted in a focus on goals and implementation strategies, not on outcomes and evaluations. Consequently, only limited information is available.

INTERVENTION HISTORY

The tax work-off program was first implemented in the Massachusetts community of Chelmsford in 1992. The Council on Aging Director modeled the program on a similar, although more limited, program in existence in Littleton, Colorado, offering a school-district tax credit to seniors who volunteered for either of the regional school districts.

The Director discussed the idea with the Chelmsford Town Counsel to obtain a legal opinion, and with the Selectmen. There were two major concerns: whether employing seniors in this way might displace unionized municipal employees, and whether the municipality would be facing increased liability issues as a result of the program. The Town Counsel ruled that the program would not increase liability because the seniors would be considered independent contractors for the purpose of this program. It was noted that the tasks designated for the program would be meaningful work that otherwise would not be accomplished. No employee would be displaced by a property tax work-off participant.

With these assurances, the tax work-off program was passed by Town Meeting with little opposition in 1992 and has been in existence ever since. The Director considers the program to be an unqualified success. Department heads are very pleased with the work of seniors, which is seen as steady, of good quality, and produced with a high level of commitment. Seniors feel proud to be able to contribute value to their community, and motivated to demonstrate their usefulness. The Director believes the program has increased interest in local government among seniors, and feedback from seniors indicates that the abatement provides a useful degree of relief from property tax pressure.

The property tax work-off program was successful enough that more than 50 other municipalities implemented versions of the program. These communities are scattered in a loose arc around Boston in eastern Massachusetts, and range in size from Lanesborough, with a population of 3,000 and a median family income of $40,000, to Framingham, with a population of 65,000 and a median family income of $53,000. The average median family income among the municipalities involved is $60,000, and the average annual property tax represents 6% of this amount. The communities vary widely in the percent of population aged 65 and older, from a low of 3% in Boxborough to a high of 19% in Belmont. The most affluent community to adopt the program is Dover, with a median family income of $103,000 and 535 seniors, or 10% of the population (Massachusetts Municipal Association, 2002). Local conditions have prompted numerous variations on the theme. The local Council on Aging commonly administers the program, but in some communities the program is administered by the Personnel Department. Most municipalities offer a $500 tax abatement or credit in exchange for 100 hours of work, but some have increased the pay rate because of concerns about matching the minimum wage. Most municipalities offer tax abatements, but one offers participating seniors a check every two weeks until a total of $525 has been earned. The recipient may do as he or she pleases with the money. This version of the program benefits elders who are not homeowners (including elders living in state-subsidized housing). It is not clear what effect this added income has on the rents assessed for subsidized apartments.

THE POLITICAL CONTEXT

When the first senior property tax work-off programs were conceived, the legal context in which they were to function was unclear. One issue of concern was the exact relationship of the program participant to the community. In working for municipal departments and receiving financial benefits, did the participants become employees? If so, were they eligible for health insurance, worker's compensation, or parity of pay with other municipal employees, and would they be subject to withholding taxes? If the participants were considered independent contractors, would they then be responsible for managing their own income tax obligations for the $500 in earned property tax credit? Could the participants truly be considered volunteers since they were receiving a financial benefit in return for their efforts? In an opinion on the tax work-off program written by Attorney Joel B. Bard of Kopelman and Page, PC, it was determined that if municipalities issued a check for the tax credit made payable to both the municipality and the participant, the program would not conflict with Massachusetts General law 59, §58, governing taxation. The Bard opinion stated that municipalities might need to provide compensation for the program that at least matches the federal minimum wage under the Fair Labor Standards Act. At the time the opinion was written, the $5 per hour rate was above the minimum wage.

Most municipalities chose to position tax work-off participants as volunteers. A $500 tax credit is not so large an incentive as to move the program from the realm of volunteerism into the world of work-for-wages. In viewing the program participants as volunteers, municipalities eliminated many of the legal complexities that might have been barriers to implementation.

A second issue was that of the reaction of unions to the creation of new, lower-cost positions in municipal departments. Susan Pope, member of the Wayland Board of Selectmen, notes that unions were concerned that the program would take work away from more highly paid union employees, with a possible loss of jobs. According to Pope, once the unions were reassured that the tasks developed for the program were tasks that the paid staff did not have time to address and that if tax work-off participants did not do the work it would simply remain incomplete, the unions were no longer resistant to the program. Pope noted that there has now been "no union objection" to the program "for years."

When it was determined that there were no legal barriers to program implementation, it was still necessary to gain consensus on the program within municipal government. Department heads, for example, needed to be educated about the benefits of the program and about the range of appropriate tasks. They needed to feel confident that the tax work-off program offered a credible source of assistance, and that participants would not require extensive orientation and training. At the same time, department heads were encouraged to develop jobs that were not just "busy work," but jobs that provided seniors with substantive opportunities to contribute valuable services to their communities.

Communities with a Town Meeting form of government needed to convince the assembly of voters to adopt and fund the program. Arguments in favor of the program were (1) its potential to retain seniors as residents (thereby avoiding the potential sale of their houses to young families with children, with the associated impact on the school budget), (2) the unfairness of forcing long-term residents to move out of the community because of inability to pay property taxes, (3) the value of the services seniors would be providing, and (4) the relatively small negative effect on total tax revenues.

POLICY OPTIONS

Strategies for strengthening the implementation of the tax work-off programs can be grouped according to three main topic areas: eligibility options, benefit options, and options to enhance returns on investment. These options are discussed in detail in the following subsections.

Eligibility Options

Eligibility options are those that broaden or restrict the class of persons deemed appropriate to participate in the tax work-off program. The goal is to provide the best fit between the provision of qualified workers for municipal departments and the provision of the tax credit benefit for the largest number of participants, while maintaining affordability for the municipality.

Age. Most tax work-off programs are open to those aged 60 and older. This eligibility limitation springs from two of the program's principle goals: to lessen the tax burden on long-term residents living on fixed incomes who might otherwise be forced to leave the community due to the rising costs of property taxes, and to retain seniors in residence both for their contributions to the diversity of the community and as a buffer against sales of their homes to families with young children, who can be expected to increase municipal expenditures for education.

The age for participation might be adjusted upward to age 65. The change could be justified because people between ages 60 and 65 can be expected to be employed full-time, and, therefore, no more in need of property tax relief than any other wage earner. A variant would be to extend eligibility to those between ages 60 and 65 if applicants can demonstrate that they are permanently retired. Adjusting age eligibility upward to 70 could be justified by noting that those most in need of property tax relief are those who have been living on fixed incomes for some period of time, during which inflation and rising taxes serve to reduce the value of private pensions and increase the cost of homeownership. Adjusting age eligibility could preserve program "slots" for those most in need. In communities where political approval of the tax work-off program is in doubt, such a change might increase the acceptability of the program to younger taxpayers. On the other hand, seniors who are employed full-time are unlikely to apply for the tax work-off program, because the task schedule would conflict with the normal hours of paid employment. In practical terms, therefore, adjusting the lower age eligibility from 60 to 65 is unlikely to have a significant effect on program enrollment.

The age for participation might also be adjusted downward for certain classes of individuals. Participants might include homeowners with permanent disabilities that preclude full-time employment. Such individuals are likely to have difficulty meeting their property tax obligations. Making it easier for them to remain in the community would preserve diversity.

Means Tests. Programs must choose whether or not to require a means test for participation. Many municipalities have no formal means tests, although an informal guideline usually indicates that where there are two equally qualified applicants for one job, the applicant in greater financial need is to be placed in the position. In practice this equivalence of skills rarely occurs. Other municipalities do require that tax work-off participants meet an income eligibility test. The exact form of this test varies with the administering body. In one community, where participation in the tax work-off program does not require homeownership, residence in a HUD-subsidized elderly housing complex is considered proof of income eligibility for the program. Another community requires that participants meet income guidelines for state subsidized Aging Services Access Point (ASAP) services. In most municipalities that require a means test, the proof of income requirements has been simplified to lighten the administrative burden on the program.

The advantages inherent in means testing the program include the assurance that the tax benefit is targeted only to those who are truly in financial need of assistance, and some assurance that the potential pool of applicants is not as numerous as all people aged 60 and older in the municipality. Means testing the program may also increase its political viability among other groups of taxpayers.

There are two major disadvantages of means testing the program. First, when participation is reserved for those seen as financially needy, the program may come to share the stigma that has damaged a similar program in Colorado. If seniors come to believe the program is only for the poor or is a form of charity, they may be reluctant to participate. Second, in accepting only those participants who qualify in terms of income, municipalities may be precluding services from seniors with valuable skills. While it would not be appropriate to assume that low-income seniors have fewer useful skills, it is still true that retired physicians, educators, and engineers may not pass the means test yet might have skills unavailable among those of lower income. In communities with no means test, highly skilled seniors with higher incomes have, in fact, been program participants.

Skill Sets. Studies have shown that using volunteers has a cost in terms of staff time. A ratio of one hour of paid staff time to about 13 hours of volunteer service is average, but the ratio varies widely (Murowski, cited in Fischer & Schaeffer, 1993, p. 132). The same study estimated the value of volunteer time is $9.33 for every $1 of paid staff time. Department heads usually do not have the resources to provide extensive on-the-job training to develop new skill sets among seniors. This is especially true given the relatively short-term nature of the work-off commitment. If the total time to be devoted to any position is 100 hours over the course of a year, it is counterproductive to allocate 25 or 30 of those hours to training.

Several municipalities have structured their tax work-off programs to match skills sought by department heads with skills available in the applicant pool in order to provide both parties the optimum work experiences. In requesting service from a tax work-off participant, department heads are seeking assistance that cannot be accomplished with paid employees given the current staffing pattern, or, in some cases, with a task that is transient in nature.

An option that might make senior participants more useful to municipal departments and strengthen and broaden the set of skills available would be to provide training outside of the work-off program itself. Program managers could assess both the skills currently available in the applicant pool and the skills being requested by department managers, to determine if there are systematic gaps. Where gaps are identified, training programs could be designed to prepare seniors for program participation. A tax work-off participant with the requisite skills could fulfill his or her service commitment by teaching those skills to other participants, for example, to train others in the use of computers and software.

An advantage to providing skill-enhancing training would be to enrich the options for program placement, thereby providing a more valuable return to community government for the tax relief provided. A second advantage would be increased utilization of senior center programs by elders who might not otherwise have participated. An unintended side effect might be the "bumping" by potential tax work-off participants of seniors who had previously been wait-listed for computer training. In communities where openings in the senior computer literacy programs are scarce, such preferential treatment for tax work-off participants might cause controversy.

Alternate Forms of Service. One limitation of many of the tax work-off programs is that seniors who are in poor physical health, yet wish to remain in their own homes, may not be capable of participating in the program. Despite barrier-free architecture and potential assistance with transportation, some seniors are simply too frail to devote 100 hours to work outside their homes. Yet these seniors may have high medical expenses and be most in need of the financial benefit the property tax work-off programs are implemented to provide.

An alternate form of service is offered in one community. Although the municipality limits tax work-off participants to one $500 benefit per year per household, it does allow husbands and wives to split the work commitment. Each member of a couple contributes 50 hours of service as a team. This may benefit municipal departments that have needs for greatly increased staffing at specific times during the year, such as when tax bills must be folded and mailed. The arrangement may also benefit couples in which one member wishes to participate but is limited because of the need for transportation or other assistance that a spouse can provide.

Benefit Options

Benefit options are those that adjust the monetary value of the tax benefit offered, the way in which the benefit is provided, or the amount of benefit available to either an individual or the group of participants taken as a whole. The goal of adjusting benefit options is to develop the optimal strategy to promote retention of resident seniors in the community by reducing their tax burdens.

Increase Pay Rate. While the tax work-off programs as currently constituted appear to be popular and at least moderately successful in providing property tax relief to seniors, there is a feeling among some participants that to be asked to provide skilled work at an hourly rate well below the wage paid to teenagers serving fast food is somehow demeaning and inappropriate. And although the tax work-off program is seen by many as a form of volunteering, it is seen by some as a poorly paid work option. Some municipalities have decided to change the rate of reimbursement to more closely match the minimum wage. Often this is done without increased municipal appropriations, funding the rate increase by reducing the number of program slots available. The end result is to provide an increased monetary benefit to fewer participants. Other municipalities have added a small amount to the $500 benefit to help offset the cost of taxes applied to the earned income.

In one community, where the program is administered by the Personnel Department, participants work 100 hours at $6.75 an hour. They are considered municipal employees, and receive checks made out in both their names and the name of the community. The volunteer aspect of the program has been downplayed, and the name has been changed to "Senior Corps" because "tax work-off" sounded like "indentured servitude," according to the Town Administrator. This program has never had a waiting list and places about 10 seniors a year with municipal departments.

In municipalities where tax on the average property assessment is in the $5,000 to $7,000 range, there is also a question about whether the $500 tax credit is enough to provide meaningful tax relief. Increasing the pay rate would have the effect of allowing participants to earn the same tax credit while working fewer hours. This strategy would address the concerns of participants about the low rate of recompense, but would have a negative effect on the amount of productive service garnered by municipal departments. Department managers might be less than enthusiastic about providing training and orientation to extremely short-term employees. Seniors might be less inclined to feel they had made an appreciable (and appreciated) contribution to their municipality if they worked far fewer hours.

Increase Total Benefit Ceiling. Increasing the rate of pay while at the same time holding the number of hours of service constant would have two advantages over increasing the pay rate alone. First, seniors who completed their 100-hour commitment would earn a higher property tax credit, boosting the ratio of relief provided by the program to the total property tax bill. Interest in program enrollment would grow, since the perceived monetary reward would be higher. Although most seniors enrolled in current programs appear to take their work commitment very seriously, it is also possible that receiving a higher rate of pay would strengthen the commitment of some. Second, the 100-hour commitment would maintain the interest and willingness of department heads to offer orientation, training, and job openings.

On the other hand, increasing the pay rate and keeping hours constant could adversely impact the program. If reducing the total number of available positions finances the additional benefits offered to participants, the greater financial benefit for some would come at the expense of others. As pay for the tax work-off program approached pay rates for unionized municipal employees, new questions of equity would arise. If a municipality can afford to pay seniors generously, it might be argued, why is it not offering full-time employees the opportunity to participate? The relatively approving attitude taken by unions toward the program could be jeopardized. The perspective of department heads might also shift as pay rates rose. The programs have created much goodwill in providing useful services for a reasonable investment. But if the pay rates approached that for regular employees, department heads might be more inclined to measure the value of service in financial terms and be dissatisfied if they felt the work provided did not match the dollars expended.

Adjust the Number of Available "Slots." Communities that want to benefit more seniors can increase the number of program positions offered. This option, of course, requires a greater total expenditure for the program, but for many municipalities this may be viable. Some communities have already expanded the number of slots available, and some plan to request additional slots.

Increasing the number of slots is the easiest way to benefit more seniors while keeping administrative duties simplified. This strategy also has the advantage of providing an increased probability of continued participation by individual seniors. Municipalities with long waiting lists for program enrollment often have a policy that dictates that a senior who participates one year is not eligible for participation the following year until all other seniors on the waiting list have been enrolled. This circumstance creates a practical barrier to providing substantive property tax relief, since the $500 credit cannot be relied on by an individual from one year to the next.

Implement a Sliding Benefit. A program that provides a rate of pay individually pro-rated and based on income would be well positioned to provide greater benefits for some seniors for the same total expenditure. Tax credits might range from $300 to $700 or more, depending on the income distribution in the pool of applicants. In choosing a lower monetary limit for this version of the program, program managers could consider the average tax bill in the community and select a lower limit designed to provide relief from a particular percentage of the bill.

This option would be appealing politically because it would allow a more substantial benefit for seniors most in need, without increasing costs to the taxpaying community. In addition, seniors could participate regardless of income, a circumstance that would go far to dispel any low-income stigma the program had acquired.

The disadvantage of this plan is that it could become cumbersome to administer, since it would require proof of income from participants. In addition, some seniors might choose not to participate if the burden of supplying documentation for the means test were too onerous.

Enhance Returns on Investment

Options that enhance returns on investment are those that vary the amount or duration of service, as well as those designed to augment the skills of participants so they may be prepared for a wider range of job openings. The goal of enhancing returns on investment is to allow the accomplishment of meaningful work for the community while maintaining overall program affordability.

Implement Skills Training for Participants. To realize the maximum return in services to the community for the dollars foregone in property tax revenues, programs must be able to supply department heads with participants who can accomplish meaningful work with relatively little on-the-job training. The advantage in providing selected skills training is that the community would receive more valuable service from participating seniors.

Adjust Service Hours. In providing the option of working more than 100 hours for a constant reimbursement rate, programs could expand the usefulness of the service to department heads. For example, a senior assigned to read aloud to elementary school children as an enrichment activity develops a relationship with the children he or she is serving. The relationship is mutually beneficial. But if the senior stops visiting the school halfway through the academic year because his or her service hour commitment has been satisfied, the smooth functioning of the reading program will be disrupted, and the benefit to the children may be decreased. Municipalities preferring to retain tax work-off participants in positions beyond 100 hours could choose to appropriate additional funds to provide additional property tax benefits. The net effect of making an adjustment to service hours is uncertain. Department heads would find an advantage in the additional hours of work, while some seniors would be reluctant to make a more lengthy commitment that might prevent seasonal travel or be difficult to manage in case of ill health.

Adjust Service Incumbency. The overall reaction of department heads to the tax work-off is quite positive. But when there has been an especially good match between a program participant and the task he or she is assigned, it is often difficult to deny that person an opportunity to return to the same job next year. For the department head, rotating incumbency means a continual need to train new workers and a loss of the ease that comes with established routines. For the participant, there is the loss of newly formed collegial relationships, and the loss of a sense of being valued and appreciated for his or her skill and competence.

Allowing an incumbent participant to return to the same position each year would negatively impact other program participants who would, by default, be competing for fewer available slots. The potential benefit for the enhanced functioning of a municipal department and the promotion of a longer-term involvement in municipal government might offset this negative impact, at least from the point of view of the community.

Reduce Bureaucratic Barriers. In the several years that tax work-off programs have been in existence, municipalities have adopted many strategies to attempt to reduce the impact of intersecting federal, state, and local tax policies. In many municipalities, the simple provision of a $500 tax credit was endangered by the idea that the money was, after all, a form of income and needed to be taxed by state and federal authorities. Some communities began to add enough dollars to the benefit amount to offset the increased tax burden.

In 2001, the Massachusetts legislature approved an outside section to the state budget as an overlay to Chapter 59 of the General Laws (section 5K) to allow municipalities to establish a "Senior Volunteer Tax Credit Program" for persons aged 60 and older. Under this amendment, the property tax credit cannot be considered wages for the purposes of taxation. The outside section does limit the amount of the reduction of property tax to $500 a year, and states that the rate of payment cannot be higher than the current Commonwealth minimum wage. Nothing in the law prohibits communities from designing programs with different parameters, but only those that abide by the provisions of the amendment are eligible for exemption from state income taxes. To date, there has been no comparable exemption from federal taxes for program participants.

The specificity of the state legislation is both its strength and its weakness. It is unambiguous in providing relief from state income taxation for compliant programs, but it leaves little room for adjusting the programs to meet local needs and circumstances. In addition, as property taxes rise at a rate of about 2.5% a year, the relative value of the fixed $500 tax credit diminishes. Proponents of the tax work-off plan could enlist the aid of senior advocates to exert pressure for revised legislations at the state level and a program-specific tax exemption at the federal level.

One administrative procedure is not universally applied, but should be adopted for participants who will be assigned to schools. Such participants should be subjected to a CORI (Criminal Offender Records Information) check to ensure that participants assigned to work with children have no convictions or pending charges that should prevent their employment in a school setting (Ellis & Noyes, 1990, p. 352).

Measurement of Program Effectiveness

The tax work-off programs have for the most part enjoyed enviable success rates. Department heads like the program because they receive valuable services without impacting their budgets. Participants like the program because it provides them with an opportunity to contribute meaningfully to their communities and experience the operation of municipal government firsthand. Taxpayers like the program because it costs little and helps preserve age diversity in the municipality. Councils on Aging like the program because it is easy to administer and helps involve seniors in activities that are a departure from the traditional senior center programming. However, most of the programs were enacted during an economic upswing. Voters might not feel so generous with tax revenue during a recession. It would be relatively easy for municipalities to reduce or eliminate funding for the program.

To demonstrate the program's value, simple data collection procedures could provide empirical evidence of a positive cost/benefit ratio. Most municipalities do not keep annual statistics on the program. At present, it is not possible to know how many individual seniors have been benefited in each municipality, how many were unable to keep their full commitment of hours, or whether characteristics of applicants for the program are causing the program inadvertently to serve some segments of the elderly community more generously than other segments. This type of information would be a useful tool in advocating for the continuance of the program.

Some municipalities conduct surveys to assess satisfaction with the program among participants, and some also measure satisfaction among department heads. Comments from participants are a way to demonstrate the lived experience of program participation. One such comment reflects the strong sense of responsibility participants bring to the program: "My goal was to perform to the best of my ability, so that we left a lasting remembrance of a task well done. Also that future candidates would be actively and proudly selected."

While statistical information would help strengthen the case that the programs are successful, the weight of anecdotal evidence is dramatic and presents a persuasive argument in favor of program continuation.

GUIDELINES FOR REPLICATION

The senior tax credit programs in Massachusetts have been successful in addressing the majority of the program's goals. They have reduced property tax burdens for participants, provided qualified workers for municipal departments at a low cost to the municipality, been the medium for accomplishment of meaningful work that otherwise would not have been attempted, and have fostered an increase of involvement in municipal government and affairs among seniors. The success of the programs in retaining senior homeowners in the community remains to be evaluated.

Recent federal emphasis on the importance of volunteer service at the local level may mean that the state and national political climate is receptive to this initiative. The low cost and ease of administration of the program will help to ease replication in other states. In developing a tax credit program, administrators should consider the following points:

- *Emphasize "service" and "volunteering."* Towns that stress the valuable service seniors are providing are successful at recruiting participants who remain committed to their task, continue with their assignment even after completing their committed hours of service, and express an enhanced feeling of connection to the community and to local government. Towns that consider the program to be a type of work-for-wages appear to have fewer potential enrollees. Framing the program from the outset as a volunteer service allows the program to be seen clearly as a demonstration of the value of seniors to the community rather than as response to a class of individuals in need of charity.
- *Reduce or eliminate means tests.* Employing a formal means test for participation appears to create a stigma of "poverty" or "charity," which becomes a negative incentive for program participation. Several towns are well served by an informal policy by which, in the case where there are two equally qualified applicants for one "slot," the applicant in greater financial need is chosen. Eliminating the means test has the added advantage of simplifying administrative procedures for program managers.
- *Institute skills training.* Formally linking computer and other skills training programs to skills development for the tax work-off program would provide incentives for increased senior participation in training, and would improve the pool of skills available for placement to benefit town departments.
- *Administer the program within the Council on Aging.* Most Massachusetts municipalities administer the senior tax work-off program within the Council on Aging (COA). The experience of those that do not seems to indicate that recruitment becomes an issue and the status of the participants is less likely to be that of a volunteer.

Councils on Aging are uniquely suited to publicizing the program to the older population, to assisting department heads in identifying tasks appropriate for participants, and to identifying and encouraging potential participants. COA directors who fear accepting the administrative burden for the program can employ a tax work-off participant to administer the program. This is an especially viable option where there is no means test, thereby eliminating confidentiality concerns.

- *Obtain federal tax relief.* At the present writing, federal taxes are still applied to the tax work-off benefit. Adopting legislation to allow the exemption of this benefit from the participant's income would simplify program administration, would result in very little lost revenue at the federal level, and would demonstrate to seniors that their service is appreciated and supported at all levels of government.
- *Measure program effectiveness.* To strengthen program management and to be able to defend the program, administrators should build in program evaluation systems. At a minimum, annual statistics should report the number of people participating in the program, the number who completed the work commitment, and the total money expended for the tax credit. In addition, department heads should be asked to evaluate the assistance provided by participants, indicate their opinions about the functioning of the program, and estimate how much they would have had to pay if a regular employee had accomplished the task.

AUTHOR NOTES

Kristin Kiesel is Director of Marketing for West Suburban Elder Services, Inc. (WSES), a private, nonprofit Aging Services Access Point and Area Agency on Aging located in Watertown, Massachusetts, which serves a client population of 3,000 elders and their families. She holds a Master's Degree in Counseling Psychology and is currently a PhD student in Gerontology at the University of Massachusetts in Boston.

Ms. Kiesel can be contacted at 20 Jeffrey Road, Wayland, MA 01778 (E-mail: kbkris@aol.com).

REFERENCES

AARP (2002). *Understanding Reverse Mortgages.* Accessed online at *http://www. aarp.org/revmort/contents/overview.html*

Bard, J. B. (1995). *Re: Proposed Senior Tax Relief Program.* Legal opinion, Kopelman and Paige, PC, Attorneys at Law, Boston, February 7.

Barlow, J., & Hainsworth, J. (2001). Volunteerism among older people with arthritis. *Ageing and Society, 21*(2), 203-212.

Brudney, J. L. (1990). *Fostering Volunteer Programs in the Public Sector: Planning, Initiating, and Managing Voluntary Activities*, San Francisco: Jossey-Bass Public Administration Series.

Cheang, M., Braun, K. L., & Sheeran, T. (2001). Encouraging volunteerism in older adults using stages of change-based strategies. *The Gerontologist*, October 15, 243.

Curley, M. (2001). Executive Director, Massachusetts Service Alliance, Boston, MA, interview by author, October 25.

Ellis, S. J., & Noyes, K. H. (1990). *By the People, A History of Americans as Volunteers*, Jossey-Bass Public Administration Series.

Fischer, L. R., & Schaeffer, K. B. (1993). *Older Volunteers: A Guide to Research and Practice*, Newbury Park, California: Sage Publications, Inc.

Fitzpatrick, K. (2001). Needham Town Administrator, Needham, MA, interview by author, November 7.

Griesel, R. (2001). Director, Sudbury Council on Aging, Sudbury, MA, interview by author, November 8.

Herzog, A. R., & House, J. S. (1991). Productive activities and aging well. *Generations, 15*, 49-54.

Jope, J. (2001). Director, Arlington Council on Aging, Arlington, MA, interview by author, October 24.

Lally, S. (2001). Director, Needham Council on Aging, Needham, MA, interview by author, October 16.

LeVan, P. (2001). Co-director, Wayland Council on Aging, Wayland, MA, interview by author.

MacNeil, L. (2001). Acting Director, Lexington Council on Aging, Lexington, MA, interview by author, November 14.

Mason, K. (2001). Information and Referral Specialist, Office on Aging, Fort Collins, Colorado, interview by author, October 15.

Massachusetts Municipal Association (2002). Accessed online at *http://www.mma.org/tango3/city_town_info/demographic.taf?fuction=form.html*

Pope, S. (2001). (Republican, Wayland), Massachusetts State Representative and Selectman, Town of Wayland, MA, interview by author.

Sheehan, J. (2001). Director, Westford Council on Aging, Westford, MA, interview by author, November 5.

Tegelaar, K. (2001). Director, Dover Council on Aging, Dover, MA, interview by author, November 21.

Town of Wayland (1998). Property Tax Work-Off Program: *Brochure*.

Walsh, M. (2001). Director, Chelmsford Council on Aging, Chelmsford, MA, interview by author, October 16.

Wilson, J., & Musik, M. (1999). The effects of volunteering on the volunteer. *Law and Contemporary Problems, 62*(4), 141-153.

Assessing State Efforts to Meet Baby Boomers' Long-Term Care Needs: A Case Study in Compensatory Federalism

Sanjay K. Pandey, PhD

Rutgers University

SUMMARY. The role of the state government and the character of federal-state relations in social policy have evolved considerably. Frank Thompson uses the phrase *compensatory federalism* to describe increased activity by state governments to make up for a diminished federal role. For compensatory federalism to work, it is essential for states to take leadership roles in key policy areas. Few studies examine whether states have risen to the challenge of compensatory federalism in social policy. This paper examines an emerging issue of great significance in social policy–challenges involved in meeting future long-term care needs for the baby boomer generation. The paper provides an in-depth case study of attempts by Maryland to meet the challenges of financing long-term care needs for the baby boomer generation. The detailed description of the agenda-setting and problem-structuring process in Maryland is followed by an analysis that uses three different frameworks to assess the policy development processes. These models are rooted in a bureaucratic politics perspective, an agenda-setting perspective and an interest group politics perspective. The paper concludes with a discussion of the limitations and possibilities of state leadership in the social policy sphere. *[Article copies available for a fee from The Haworth Document Delivery Service: 1-800-HAWORTH. E-mail address: <getinfo@haworthpressinc.com> Website: <http://www.HaworthPress.com> © 2002 by The Haworth Press, Inc. All rights reserved.]*

[Haworth co-indexing entry note]: "Assessing State Efforts to Meet Baby Boomers' Long-Term Care Needs: A Case Study in Compensatory Federalism." Pandey, Sanjay K. Co-published simultaneously in *Journal of Aging & Social Policy* (The Haworth Press, Inc.) Vol. 14, No. 3/4, 2002, pp. 161-179; and: *Devolution and Aging Policy* (ed: Francis G. Caro, and Robert Morris) The Haworth Press, Inc., 2002, pp. 161-179. Single or multiple copies of this article are available for a fee from The Haworth Document Delivery Service [1-800-HAWORTH, 9:00 a.m. - 5:00 p.m. (EST). E-mail address: getinfo@haworthpressinc.com].

KEYWORDS. Devolution, federalism, Medicaid, state health policy, long-term care, baby boomers

INTRODUCTION

The last two decades of the twentieth century witnessed significant shifts in the relative roles of federal and state governments in the social policy arena. The federal government's dominant role in health and social policy was eroded by sustained federal budget deficits through much of this period. Worsening fiscal crises–combined with the maze of inter-governmental rules and regulations frustrating programmatic innovation at lower levels of government–prompted calls for reforms to put state governments in the driver seat. In the aftermath of the failure of the Clinton health reform efforts in 1994, the federal government ceded much control over health policy initiatives to state governments (Thompson, 2001). While there is some debate on whether these changes putting states at the helm are permanent, there is little disagreement regarding the enhanced role of the states (Alt & Marzotto, 1999; Leichter, 1996; Nathan, 1993; Rich & White, 1996).[1]

Assessments of state governments' capacity to assume a leadership role in addressing vexing social policy issues, however, evoke both optimism and skepticism (Bloksberg, 1989; Leichter, 1996; Morris, Caro, & Hansan, 1998). Leichter (1996), for instance, rates state governments highly for their willingness and accomplishments in addressing knotty health policy issues. Evidence of significant accomplishments by state-level policymakers is provided by other scholars as well (e.g., Oliver & Paul-Shaheen, 1997). Yet others take issue with the hopeful and purposeful images conjured up by Justice Brandeis's phrase describing states as "laboratories of democracy" and underscore the inevitability and indispensability of federal leadership in social policy (Sparer & Brown, 1996; Thompson, 2001).

This paper examines whether state governments can make up for the lack of federal leadership on a social policy issue. To borrow a phrase from Thompson (1998), the question may be framed as follows: What are the prospects for *compensatory federalism*? The compensatory federalism thesis suggests that when government institutions at one level fail to address an important policy issue, corresponding institutions at another level rise up to the challenge and provide the necessary leadership and guidance (Thompson, 1998). We assess compensatory federalism by examining how state-level policy processes are addressing future long-term care needs of baby boomers.[2] Although the public-at-large pays little attention to long-term care, the oncoming "demographic tidal wave" of baby boomer retirees is likely to increase greatly the demand for long-term care services and transform this issue into an important public policy concern.

In studying the performance of compensatory federalism, we use a case-study approach focusing on state-level policy development. While a case-study approach has its limitations, especially with respect to generalizability of findings, it is appropriate, given the purposes of this study. Studying state-level processes requires generating in-depth, extensive, and contextual knowledge about unique events; purposes that are best served by a case study research design (Yin, 1994). Thus, this paper assesses the potential of compensatory federalism by describing and examining the processes by which the state of Maryland pursued and developed its *Outreach Empowerment Campaign*, an effort directed at exploring and meeting future long-term care needs. To construct the case history, we draw upon extensive publicly disseminated documentation on the Outreach Empowerment Campaign.[3] No key informant interviews were necessary because the author has conducted policy analytic work focusing on state health policy issues in Maryland for several years. This firsthand experience with Maryland health policy issues provides the supplemental knowledge base necessary for creating the case history.

While detailed and accurate description is essential, it is even more important to provide plausible models to explain the unfolding of events in a case study. Not only are these models helpful in understanding the dynamics of compensatory federalism in this case, but they also may provide guidelines for understanding workings of similar processes in less familiar settings. We propose three models to explain the outcomes of the Maryland policy development processes; these models are rooted in a bureaucratic politics perspective, an agenda-setting perspective, and an interest group politics perspective. The remainder of the paper is organized in the following manner. First, we provide a description of the overall context of health care reforms in Maryland. Next, an in-depth description of the Maryland Outreach Empowerment Campaign is provided. This description is followed by a summary overall assessment of the Campaign. The progression of events in the Outreach Empowerment Campaign is explained using the three perspectives identified earlier. The paper concludes with some thoughts on the potential of compensatory federalism and state leadership.

MARYLAND HEALTH REFORMS IN THE 1990s:
FISCAL CRISES ENGENDER PROGRAMMATIC INNOVATIONS

The pace and scope of health reforms in Maryland increased sharply in the wake of the failure of Clinton health reform efforts in 1994 (Oliver, 1998; Oliver & Oliver, 1998). Providing for future long-term care needs of baby boomers emerged as a subsidiary theme in the comprehensive reforms proposed by Maryland's Department of Health and Mental Hygiene. Policy development to meet baby boomers' long-term care needs required attention to several issues such as defining the nature of the looming fiscal crisis, obtaining public input, and raising public awareness. These activities were carried out under the rubric of a project titled "The Outreach Empowerment Campaign." This project received institutional leadership from the Department of Health and Mental Hygiene (DHMH). Much of the technical and operational assistance to DHMH was provided by the Center for Health Program Development and Management (CHPDM), based at the University of Maryland, Baltimore County.

Since the Campaign was a small part of a much larger reform effort, it is important to know the context and the relevant details of the larger reform effort. The rapid growth in Medicaid budgets during the 1990s became a matter of concern for most states, prompting the use of descriptors like "budget buster" (Boyd, 1998). Medicaid expenses continued to rise in Maryland, comprising an ever greater proportion of the state budget, reaching nearly two billion dollars in state fiscal year 1994 (Oliver, 1998). Few things are as powerful as a budget crisis in stimulating programmatic innovations. Maryland, much like other states, sought ways to contain growth in Medicaid expenses (Daniels, 1998; Oliver & Oliver, 1998).

Maryland was one of the first states to enroll most of its Medicaid beneficiaries in a primary care case management program named Maryland Access to Care (MAC) in 1991. By increasing payments for physician visits by nearly 50% and intensive outreach efforts, the MAC program sought to provide a medical home for Medicaid beneficiaries (Schoenman, Evans, & Schur, 1997). Maryland's continued efforts to look for ways to contain costs led to the genesis of the High Cost User Initiative (HCUI). This program targeted Medicaid patients with high levels of inpatient recidivism. It reduced readmissions by linking these patients to a case manager who facilitated access to health and social service providers (LoBianco, Mills, & Moore, 1996; Stuart & Weinreich, 1998).

The course of Maryland health reform was profoundly influenced by two events in 1994, the first (as noted earlier) being the failure of Clinton reforms, and the second, the change in state health policy leadership.[4] The leadership change dramatically affected the scope and pace of reforms with the new administration's view of health reforms representing a paradigm shift, from incremental programmatic improvements to comprehensive system-wide reforms (Oliver, 1998). The DHMH proposal for comprehensive health care reform, conceived and developed under the new leadership, led to the passage of Senate Bill 750 after due deliberation and modification on the last day of 1996 legislative session (Oliver, 1998).

The Senate Bill 750 addressed reform of the Medicaid programs serving the non-elderly and the elderly quite differently. For the non-elderly Medicaid population (composed of families and children and disabled beneficiaries not in need of long-term care), the reform proposal presented a full-blown outline for phasing in all the beneficiaries into managed care as well as a complete redesign of the mental health system serving poor and uninsured state residents. In contrast to the extensive, detailed, and specific reform efforts directed at non-elderly Medicaid beneficiaries, Senate Bill 750 proposed a detailed study of managed long-term care initiatives. Specifically, it directed the DHMH Secretary to establish a Long-Term Managed Care Advisory Committee with a representative membership to "advise on development of a managed care proposal for the Medicaid long-term care population."

Although the authorizing legislation was focused on studying expansion of managed care to the Medicaid long-term care population, it also provided some latitude for exploring related issues by calling for the creation of a Long-Term Care Managed Care Technical Advisory Committee. The Outreach Empowerment Campaign, a project aimed at understanding the nature of the fiscal challenge posed by long-term care needs of aging baby boomers and providing public education, grew out of subsequent deliberations and recommendations of this technical advisory committee.

MARYLAND'S OUTREACH EMPOWERMENT CAMPAIGN: A CHRONOLOGY AND DESCRIPTION

While other aspects of the reform effort were linked to specific programmatic areas under the Department's ambit, meeting future long-term care financing needs emerged as a "stand-alone" issue. Thus, two key goals of the Outreach Empowerment Campaign–defining the fiscal challenge posed by baby boomers' future long-term care needs and raising public awareness–did not have strong ties to specific programs or populations served by DHMH.[5] The beginning of the Outreach Empowerment Campaign (the "Campaign" hereafter) was fairly innocuous (see Table 1 for a chronology of key events). Senate Bill 750 directed the DHMH Secretary to study the feasibility of various managed care options for long-term care populations covered by Maryland Medicaid. The legislation authorized the creation of a 15-member Long-Term Managed Care Advisory Committee with broad representation and chartered it to study eligibility, benefits, financing, and implementation issues surrounding long-term managed care. There was no mention of the need for efforts to understand the nature and scope of potential fiscal challenges posed by baby boomers' future long-term care needs.

So, how did this process result in the creation of the Campaign that conducted an extensive study of baby boomers' future long-term care needs? Although the authorizing legislation did not explicitly address this issue, it provided for a consultative process involving public meetings across the state. With staff support from DHMH and CHPDM, the fifteen-member Long-Term Managed Care Advisory Committee made up of providers, consumer advocates, legislators, and agency representatives met almost weekly through the summer of 1996, hearing testimony from a variety of groups (Long-Term Managed Care Advisory Committee, 1996). By mid-fall of 1996 when the committee was beginning to wind up its efforts for a November 1 report to the DHMH Secretary, it had heard testimony from academic experts, provider groups, agency staff, consumer advocates as well as the general public. In a wide-ranging report on different long-term care populations and managed care options, two recommendations at the very end highlighted the need for a public education campaign on future long-term care needs. One of these recommended development of incentives to promote purchase of long-term care insurance; the other recommendation was, "Funding should be set aside for an ongoing state-sponsored educational campaign to the general population, their risks for needing long term-care, costs of long-term care. . . . The campaign must stress the financial reality of decreasing resources for Medicaid coverage of long term-care" (Long-Term Managed Care Advisory Committee, 1996, p. 52).

Given the thrust of the DHMH-led effort to explore and develop managed care options for long-term care populations served by Medicaid, it would have been relatively easy for DHMH to set aside the call for public education. However, Secretary Wasserman put great emphasis

TABLE 1. Time Line and Milestones for the Outreach Empowerment Campaign

Time	Milestone	Key Outcome
April 1996	Passage of Senate Bill 750	Formation of Long-Term Managed Care Advisory Committee
November 1996	Advisory Committee completes report	Recommended development of programs to educate the public about long-term care
January 1997	Secretary's report to the Maryland General Assembly regarding Long-Term Managed Care Advisory Committee	Secretary recommends symposium to plan a "broad-based educational program"
Summer 1998	Symposium conducted at University of Maryland, Baltimore County	Identified goals for the educational program and recommended methods
1998-1999	Publicizing the program and obtaining support from various public and private institutions	Presentation to the State Interagency Committee on Aging Services, various area agencies on aging, etc.
2000		Continuance of presentations and search for further funding

on the public education campaign in a series of meetings conducted prior to reporting to Maryland General Assembly in 1997, going so far as to commission the planning and development of a public education campaign: "Today, individuals protect themselves and their families, to the best of their ability, against the costs of acute illness. They similarly need to plan to protect themselves against the costs of long-term care" (Wasserman, 1997). The first step in development of this broad public education campaign was the convening of a symposium to consider the effects of long-term care on families and communities, providing accurate information on long-term care, and publicizing the importance of long-term care insurance to opinion leaders.

The symposium was convened a year and a half later and was organized by CHPDM acting on behalf of DHMH. With adequate time for planning, CHPDM was able to organize a symposium with over 450 attendees (CHPDM, 1998a). After a morning plenary session, the symposium had a working session in the afternoon on four themes: health promotion, independent living, insurance-based options to pay for long-term costs, and non-insurance-based strategies to cover long-term care costs (CHPDM, 1998a). The symposium uncovered several limitations of insurance-based strategies, such as the public's lack of trust regarding long-term care insurance, lack of affordable insurance options, and unavailability of reliable information. Interestingly, the symposium also brought to light several non-insurance-based strategies such as reverse mortgages and financial planning. Planning for a "spectrum of services" on aging and incorporating personal health planning as a means to obviate future long-term care needs also emerged as themes (CHPDM, 1998a).

The extensive and extended consultation period, thus, led to novel ideas for a public education campaign on future long-term care needs. Subsequent to the symposium, a business plan for implementing the Campaign was developed that outlined an underlying philosophy, goals, and outcomes and a time line for implementation (CHPDM, 1998b). The underlying philosophy for the Campaign had three key elements: using education to empower consumers, relying on public-private partnerships, and concentrating resources on defined populations (CHPDM, 1998b; Kaelin, 1999). By providing accurate and timely information to Maryland citizens on long-term care, the Campaign hoped to help Maryland adults exercise personal responsibility in planning to meet their long-term care needs.

Following development of consensus on key thematic issues for the Campaign, a number of presentations were made by the campaign to various state agencies including the State Interagency Committee on Aging Services. By presenting the plan to key stakeholders in the executive and legislative circles, the Campaign hoped to obtain a "firm commitment" to the goals and methods of the campaign (CHPDM, 1998b). Over the next year, Campaign philosophy, goals, and methods were presented to several key policymakers at both the statewide and local levels (CHPDM, 1998b).

OVERALL ASSESSMENT AND ANALYSIS OF LIMITATIONS OF THE MARYLAND CAMPAIGN: THREE POSSIBLE EXPLANATIONS

One of the more remarkable aspects of the Campaign was that the ideas motivating it emerged spontaneously through public consultation. With strong support from the highest level in Maryland health policy leadership, namely Secretary Wasserman, the Campaign's accomplishments on two fronts were significant. First, it was successful in "fleshing out" and vetting the complex set of issues surrounding baby boomers' future long-term care needs. The Campaign brought into sharp relief limitations of Medicaid reform and private insurance. It also highlighted alternate financial and health-based approaches for long-term care planning. Second, the Campaign was successful in communicating this message statewide to a select audience. DHMH, the lead agency, assisted by CHPDM, was also able to disseminate this message to a wide body of governmental and non-governmental actors in the state. This is the point at which the Campaign seems to have hit a *cul de sac*.

The public education component did not advance beyond this group of corporate entities to the wider target audience of baby boomer residents of the state. Relatedly, the Campaign was not able to enlist specific support from agencies other than those providing staff support (DHMH and CHPDM). In sum, the key contribution of the Campaign from a policymaking perspective had to do with insertion of some new ideas regarding baby boomers' future long-term care needs in the long-term care policy community in Maryland (Kingdon, 1984).

A more recent update from DHMH on the Campaign noted that, "A business plan for the campaign was developed, and funding is being sought. Meetings are being held with public and private leaders and stakeholders across the state to discuss the Campaign's implementation. CHPDM is developing an educational program for outreach, including a Web site, which should be ready by Fall of 2000" (DHMH, 2000). An examination of the CHPDM Web site, at different times from 2000 to 2002, indicated that the site cannot be described as an "educational Web site" to spread the Campaign's message. Additionally, a comparison of the Campaign time line (Table 1) with other aspects of comprehensive reforms showed that implementation was much farther along for other projects. For example, the Medicaid managed care program, HealthChoice, demonstration projects on long-term care, a case management program for vulnerable Medicaid beneficiaries have accomplished much and have been operational for several years (DHMH, 2000; Leeds, 2000; Pandey et al., 2000; Weiner et al., 1998).

Thus, it is reasonable to infer that despite initial successes, the Campaign seems to have fizzled with no tangible programmatic results. Yet the policy development processes entailed in the Campaign can provide valuable lessons and guidelines about conditions under which state leadership can be effective. We employ three different analytical perspectives: a bureaucratic politics perspective, an agenda-setting perspective, and an interest group politics perspective. After the analyses, we discuss the value of the lessons learned from the Campaign.

Context for Policy Development:
Key State Agencies, Competing Policy Priorities,
and Bureaucratic Politics

Maryland, like most states, has a number of agencies that have an effect on long-term care policies, programs, and services. Key agencies that have impacts on long-term care in Maryland are the Department of Health and Mental Hygiene, Department of Aging, Department of Human Resources, Department of Budget and Management, Department of Housing and Community Development, and the Governor's Office on Individuals with Disabilities. These agencies perform a variety of functions related to long-term care including operation of home care programs, provision of social services, home financing and modification, information clearinghouse, and policy coordination on specific long-term care issues.

DHMH is a large state health agency with primary responsibility for policy development and program operations in three key areas, namely Medicaid, public health, and mental health. The Medicaid program operated by DHMH spent nearly $1.24 billion dollars on long-term care in 1999 (Leeds, 2000). Much of this spending was either to support existing long-term care programs or for development of new programs in three areas: enhancement of HCBS waivers, development of consumer-directed care models, and development of care systems that integrate long-term care and acute care (Leeds, 2000). With most of the operational effort taken up by these programs, there was little support within DHMH for a future-oriented educational campaign on long-term care targeted at the population-at-large. Further, the DHMH-led effort failed to obtain more than nominal cooperation from other state government agencies responsible for long-term care services.

The other lead agency in the Campaign, CHPDM, a university-based contractor, was not so constrained by its mission as the line agencies in the state government. Yet, there was little CHPDM could do autonomously.[6] CHPDM was created as a joint venture between DHMH and the University of Maryland, Baltimore County, in 1994. Since its inception as a direct provider of case management services, CHPDM has transformed into an organization that is able to provide support on a variety of policy research and program support activities (Oliver, 1998; Oliver & Oliver, 1998).

During the devolution heyday in the 1990s when the state legislature was unwilling to approve additional personnel for DHMH, the Department was able to build this capacity by contracting out to the University of Maryland, Baltimore County (Oliver, 1998). However, CHPDM does not have an autonomous legislatively-chartered mission. Its primary role is one of providing technical assistance to DHMH. Thus, though CHPDM was in a position to provide staff support to the Campaign, it could not proceed to rally support in executive and legislative circles like a typical mission-based agency.

From the perspective of the Campaign, 1999 was a signal year that brought about a turnover of health policy leadership that had overseen health reforms since 1994 at DHMH. When the new health policy leadership took over at DHMH in 1999, several years of budget surpluses had rendered somewhat unnecessary the need to pursue policy development efforts such as the Campaign to meet future financing challenges. More pressing for this new administration was the need to address the operational problems being faced by the centerpiece of health reforms, the Medicaid managed care program (HealthChoice), serving nearly 400,000 beneficiaries in Maryland. There were high-profile errors in the risk-adjusted capitation system for HealthChoice; keeping the managed care organizations interested in continued participation posed a challenge, and there were few visible indicators of cost savings or quality improvements in the HealthChoice program (Garland, 1999; Salganik, 2001; Salganik, 2000; Sugg, 2000; Wheeler, 1999).

If there is one maxim in public policy with which few would quibble, it is that "the squeaky wheel gets the grease" (Bardach, 2000). Thus, it is not surprising that the new DHMH leadership, which probably had a somewhat different set of policy priorities, attended to the immediate operational needs thrust upon them by the HealthChoice program and not to furthering the Campaign aimed at stemming future long-term care expenses.

Agenda-Setting and Problem-Structuring Processes in the Outreach Empowerment Campaign

The failure of extensive and extended efforts by the Campaign to elicit broad and sustained public participation, one of its avowed goals, deserves some scrutiny. One of the most sophisticated models of agenda-setting processes has been advanced by Cobb and Elder (1972), and we will use this model for analyzing the progress of the Campaign. This model is helpful for obtaining an understanding of how an issue is defined and the processes by which it becomes salient to the public at large. According to Cobb and Elder (1972), issues are created through a dynamic process of interaction between a "triggering device" and an "initiator." A triggering device provides an opportunity for the initiator to spark public deliberation about an issue.

The failure of Clinton health reforms and extended budget shortfalls at the state and federal levels for several years, together with the ascendence of 104th Congress that favored devolution to the states in the social policy arena, served as the triggering devices. Policymakers at the state level, especially those in charge of the Medicaid program (the largest payer for long-term expenses), viewed the prospect of huge potential expenses for baby boomers' long-term care needs with limited help from the federal government as a major risk. Therefore, DHMH (aided by CHPDM) served as the initiator for bringing the issue of financing future long-term care needs of baby boomers to public notice.

From the perspective of the initiators, the public education campaign may have been a pro-active effort to mobilize the public as well as other significant public and private actors to cooperate in exploring different ways of helping the initiators cope with this potential liability. Although the initiators failed to drive this issue forward, making it a salient issue for other actors, the involvement of a large number of groups helped bring out the complexity and multi-dimensional nature of the problem posed by the aging of baby boomers.

Cobb and Elder (1972) use the term "systemic agenda" to describe legitimate matters for public concern, issues that receive full public consideration. Cobb and Elder stipulate that an issue needs to satisfy three criteria to become part of the systemic agenda: widespread awareness of the issue, public concern regarding action, and falling within the legitimate jurisdiction of an agency. Furthermore, Cobb and Elder assert that "the quicker an issue can be converted into an emotional issue, the greater the likelihood that it will gain public visibility " (Cobb & Elder, 1972, p. 124).

Viewed through the models of issue expansion proposed by Cobb and Elder, the gradual (almost glacial) pace at which baby boomers' long-term care needs are likely to become manifest worked against it. Also, the issue lacked the three key characteristics Cobb and Elder identify as pre-requisite for expansion, namely widespread awareness, clamor for public action, and assurance regarding jurisdiction of the initiating agency. While health care was very much in the public consciousness and there was credible call for action, few considered the issue of long-term care as an issue in its own right. Even fewer readily made the connection between the aging of baby boomers and the need for long-term care and its implications for public budgets. When this is combined with other competing policy priorities, it is not surprising that this issue did not expand to become part of the systemic agenda.

Interest Group Politics:
Middle Class Entitlement in the Medicaid Program

While viewing the failure of the long-term education campaign itself by examining it in light of agenda-setting models is valuable, considering the campaign as one part of a large reform package provides further insights. As noted in an earlier section, the emergence of the new federalism and long-standing fiscal uncertainty prompted DHMH in Maryland to scrutinize closely health care expenditures. The result of this close examination was a comprehensive reform package that was to be implemented in two phases, with many of the reforms pertaining to long-term care to be pursued in the later phase. In light of the fact that expenditures related to long-term care are larger and growing more quickly than other parts of the Medicaid budget, at first glance the phasing of the reform effort seems backward (Leeds, 2000; Oliver, 1998; Stuart & Weinreich, 1998). This "backward ordering" is not surprising if the reforms are viewed through the lens of interest group politics.

Several scholars, notably Grogan (1991; 1993), have argued that middle class entitlements in the Medicaid program enjoy strong and effective political support. Historically, policymakers have been more responsive to organized interest groups (Anton, 1989; Oliver & Dowell, 1994; Grogan, 1993). Provider groups as well as potential beneficiaries of long-term care services are better organized as compared with other Medicaid stakeholders. This strong political support is reflected in both the absolute amount and rate of growth in long-term care expenditure. The rate of growth in expenditures for elderly and disabled recipients has increased more quickly than that for other Medicaid groups (Burwell & Rymer, 1987; Grogan, 1993).

From an interest group politics perspective, the reform-package proposed in 1995 by the DHMH contained two types of provisions. The first kind, directed at politically powerless interest groups, were more definitive, more detailed, and were directed at making significant changes to the existing system (Pandey et al., 2000; Weiner et al., 1998). Contrasted with definitive proposals targeting politically powerless groups, reform proposals regarding long-term care programs and policies were less explicit and provided for greater public involvement. Moreover, in addition to slating long-term care reforms for later phases of the reform process, issues such as long-term care planning for baby boomers may have served as a dirigible to detract attention from other significant long-term care reform issues. By focusing on distal long-term care financing needs of baby boomers, more proximal issues, such as financing long-term care for the near-poor elderly, issues over which DHMH had clear jurisdiction, may not have received adequate attention.

DISCUSSION

The 1990s have been dubbed "the decade of devolution." National governments all over the globe rushed to transfer responsibility to state governments, often with uncertain results, leading one observer to characterize devolution as a "leap in the dark" (Lomas, 1999). *Compensatory federalism* offers a more optimistic perspective on devolution. According to Thompson (1998, 51), ". . . compensatory federalism asserts that policy retreat at one level of the federal system often spurs new activity at another level." Although skepticism regarding state capacity to address pressing social policy issues is quite common, there is a growing recognition that states are increasingly spearheading significant reform efforts (Alt & Marzotto, 1999; Leichter, 1996; Oliver & Paul-Shaheen, 1997). As Leichter (1996, p. 17) points out, state leadership in successful reform efforts is discernible in states as diverse as Hawaii, Maine, Oregon, and Texas, where "policymakers have shown extraordinary innovativeness and sensitivity in dealing with some of our most intractable health related problems."

What is it that makes some states more successful than others in addressing key social policy issues? The diversity across states, in governance mechanisms and political cultures, is a source of challenge in discovering universal patterns. However, in-depth case studies like the one presented in this article offer a valuable means for understanding the policymaking processes at the state level. The case study approach used in this paper is appropriate, despite limitations of generalizability and external validity. Indeed, cumulation of findings from studies like this (e.g., Hackey, 1998; Sparer, 1996) can provide insight into the limitations and possibilities of state leadership on social policy issues in different institutional environments.

This study demonstrates that more than mere administrative prowess is necessary for states to make significant policy accomplishments. States must provide their own "motive force" by fostering policy development processes that are autonomous in agenda setting and insightful in problem structuring. The current study offers lessons regarding issue identification and progression in state policymaking circles. For compensatory federalism to deliver the results, states must create institutional mechanisms for identifying and fostering the development of new ideas. Often, policymaking at the state level is reactive, responding to the latest changes at the federal level (Oliver, 1998; Sparer, 1996). Furthermore, policymaking at the state level tends to rely on a limited set of actors for new ideas (e.g., professional administrators, legislative analysts). Bringing other stakeholders into policy development process, as in the public deliberation process on long-term care initiated by DHMH, can help inject new ideas. However, support from top political leadership is essential for these ideas to flourish, as is evident from this case study.

Despite the extended period of attention to future long-term care needs of baby boomers (see Table 1 for time lines), no new policies and programs were enacted. The three models discussing the dynamics of issue progression provide insight into the reasons behind stalling of the policy development efforts. First, as the agenda-setting perspective makes clear, the inherent dimensions of a policy issue have a significant impact on the progression of policy development efforts. Second, the interest group politics perspective suggests that the most important lesson for state-level policymaking leadership is the value of the ability to work successfully with interest groups. Policymakers's ability to articulate clearly the stakes for different interest groups has the potential to motivate self-interested action consistent with broader policy goals. To some extent, the Campaign's inability to proceed beyond a certain point may be due to the fact that DHMH was not able to provide well articulated rationale and motivation for other governmental and non-governmental actors.

Finally, the analysis from a bureaucratic politics perspective points to difficulties state agencies may face in policy development in contested or unclaimed policy domains. In addition to other activities necessary for policy development, the focal agency needs to build a consensus around its preferred perspective and in the process gain the necessary legitimacy to pursue further action. Clearly, pursuing the objective of meeting future long-term care expenses for the population at large necessitated the involvement of a large number of external stakeholders. An alternate approach could have focused on devising strategies to meet future long-term care expenses for the poor and the near-poor. While not meeting the overarching goal in one fell swoop, this strategy could be productive in two ways. First, by restricting its focus to groups for which DHMH already had responsibility for design and operation of programs, the task of creating new programs and policies would have been considerably easier. Second, these accomplishments could become the first steps in a sequence of steps through which these programs could be expanded to the larger population.

How can the analysis in this paper be used in a productive manner by state policymakers? The three models may serve as analytical tools to assess the limitations to and possibilities of policymaking leadership at the state level. Assessments like these, rather than ideological preferences or prevailing attitudes on federalism, can be used to drive state-level policy development efforts in policy domains devoid of federal leadership.

NOTES

1. The character of new federalism that grew out of the 1980s and 1990s, with its emphasis on state leadership, stands in sharp contrast to federal-state relations in an earlier era of some ferment. Sundquist and Davis (1969, p. 4) describe the dominant federal role in federal-state relations during the 1960s in the following words: "The program remains a federal program; as a matter of administrative convenience, the federal government executes the program through state or local governments rather than through its own field offices, but the motive force is federal, with states and communities assisting, rather than the other way around."

2. The fiscal challenge posed by the aging population is one that neither the public nor existing public programs are prepared to deal with (Morris, Caro, & Hansan, 1998). Medicare provides for extremely limited long-term care coverage. The prospect of federal initiatives to meet this emerging need is dim. Medicare reform efforts over the last several years have failed to make modest strides in the direction of providing incremental reforms such as pharmaceutical coverage; therefore, expecting radical redesign of the program to build in coverage for long-term care is not realistic. Similarly, the extant burden of providing support for a public long-term care system by the Medicaid program is so heavy, that it is not reasonable to expect the Medicaid program to expand long-term care coverage.

3. As of March 2002, most of this material was available on the Web site http://www.umbc.edu/chpdm/ltc.htm.

4. In 1994, Martin Wasserman took the oath of office as Secretary of the Department of Health and Mental Hygiene. Dr. Wasserman served till 1999 and was succeeded in this position by Dr. Georges Benjamin.

5. To be precise, the Campaign does not use the specific term "baby boomer"; instead, the target population is defined as "adults over the age of 40."

6. Organizations like CHPDM are going to be increasingly important in state policy development efforts. Despite the lack of line responsibilities, such organizations play a pivotal role, defining and elaborating on policy alternatives.

AUTHOR NOTES

Sanjay K. Pandey is Assistant Professor and Director for the Health Care Management and Policy Concentration of the MPA degree in the Department of Public Policy and Administration, Rutgers University. His research and teaching interests focus on public management and health policy. His research has been accepted in journals such as *Social Science & Medicine, Journal of Policy Analysis & Management* and *Journal of Public Administration Research & Theory.*

Professor Pandey can be contacted at Rutgers University, Department of Public Policy and Administration, 401 Cooper Street, Camden, NJ 08102 (E-mail: skpandey@camden.rutgers.edu).

The author gratefully acknowledges insightful comments on an earlier version of the paper by David Frankford, Robert Morris, Sheela Tiwary, and an anonymous reviewer that have greatly strengthened the paper. The article also benefitted from interactions and exchanges with former colleagues in the Maryland health policy community.

This work was supported in part by partial summer support from the Center for State Health Policy at Rutgers University in the summer of 2001. Naturally, the support from the above named parties does not necessarily imply an endorsement of the opinions and interpretations in the article.

REFERENCES

Alt, P. M., & Marzotto, T. (1999). Federalism and health care. In Kilpatrick, A. O. and Johnson, J. A. (Eds.), *Handbook of Health Administration and Policy*. New York: Marcel Dekker.

Anton, T. (1989). *American Federalism and Public Policy*. Philadelphia, PA: Temple University Press.

Bardach, E. (2000). *A Practical Guide for Policy Analysis: The Eightfold Path to More Effective Problem Solving*. Chatham, NJ: Chatham House Publishing.

Bloksberg, L. M. (1989). Intergovernmental relations: Change and continuity. *Journal of Aging and Social Policy, 1,* 11-36.

Boyd, D. J. (1998). Medicaid devolution: A fiscal perspective. In Thompson, F. J. and DiIulio, J. J. (Eds.), *Medicaid and Devolution: A View from the States*. Washington, DC: Brookings Institution Press.

Burwell, B. O., & Rymer, M. P. (1987). Trends in Medicaid eligibility. *Health Affairs, 6,* 30-45.

Center for Health Program Development and Management (1998a). A Symposium on Personal and Public Responsibilities in Meeting Long-Term Care Needs. (Available at *http://www.umbc.edu/chpdm/sympsumm.htm*; Access Date: June 2001.)

Center for Health Program Development and Management (1998b). "Outreach Empowerment Campaign for Individual Long-Term Care Campaign: Presented to Interagency Committee on Aging Services." December 14, 1998, University of Maryland, Baltimore County.

Cobb, R. W., & Elder, C. D. (1972). *Participation in American Politics: The Dynamics of Agenda Building*. Boston, MA: Allyn and Bacon, Inc.

Daniels, M. R. (1998). *Medicaid Reform and the American States: Case Studies on the Politics of Managed Care*. Westport, CT: Auburn House.

Department of Health and Mental Hygiene (2000). Maryland Medicaid Reform-Phase II–Long-Term Care Status As of June 15, 2000. (Available at *http://www.dhmh.state.md.us/hsaea/html/phase2upd.htm*; Access Date: June 2001.)

Garland, G. (1999). "Poor's care below par, study says." *Baltimore Sun,* August 28.

Grogan, C. M. (1993). Federalism and health care reform. *American Behavioral Scientist, 36*(6), 741-759.

Grogan, C. M. (1991). *A Political Theory to Explain the Variation in State Medicaid Policy*. Ph.D. Dissertation, University of Minnesota.

Hackey, R. B. (1998). *Rethinking Health Care Policy: The New Politics of State Regulation*. Washington, DC: Georgetown University Press.

Kaelin, J. J. (1999). "Emerging payer systems for senior health care: Mind, body, money." Presentation at the 17th Annual Conference of the Maryland Gerontological Association, May 17, 1999; Baltimore, Maryland.

Kingdon, J. W. (1984). *Agendas, Alternatives, and Public Policies.* New York: HarperCollins.

Leeds, M. (2000). "Overview of the Medicaid Long-Term Care System in Maryland." Presentation made to the Medicaid Community Access Task Force, October 24. (Available at *www.dhmh.state.md.us*; Access Date: June 20, 2001.)

Leichter, H. M. (1996). State governments and their capacity for health care reform. In Rich, R. F. & White, W. D. (Eds.), *Health Policy, Federalism and the American States.* Washington, DC: The Urban Institute Press.

LoBianco, M. S., Mills, M. E., & Moore, H. W. (1996). A model for case management of high cost Medicaid users. *Nursing Economics, 14,* 303-307.

Lomas, J. (1999). The evolution of devolution: What does the community want? In Drache, D. and Sullivan, T. (Eds.), *Market Limits in Health Reform: Public Success, Private Failure.* New York: Routledge.

Long-Term Managed Care Advisory Committee (1996). *Findings and Recommendations for Long-Term Managed Care in Maryland.* November 1. (Available at *http://www.umbc.edu/chpdm/ltc.htm*; Access Date: June 2001.)

Morris, R., Caro, F. G., & Hansan, J. E. (1998). *Personal Assistance: The Future of Home Care.* Baltimore, MD: The Johns Hopkins University Press.

Nathan, R. P. (1993). The role of the states in American federalism. In Van Horn, C. E. (Ed.), *The State of the States,* 2nd Edition. Washington, DC: CQ Press.

Oliver, T. R. (1998). The collision of economics and politics in Medicaid managed care: Reflections on the course of reform in Maryland. *The Milbank Quarterly, 76*(1), 59-101.

Oliver, T. R., & Dowell, E. B. (1994). Interest groups and health reform: Lessons from California. *Health Affairs, 13*(1), 123-141.

Oliver, T. R., & Oliver, K. A. (1998). Managed care or managed politics? Medicaid reforms in Maryland. In Daniels, M. R. (Ed.), *Medicaid Reform and the American States: Case Studies on the Politics of Managed Care.* Westport, CT: Auburn House.

Oliver, T. R., & Paul-Shaheen, P. (1997). Translating ideas into actions: Entrepreneurial leadership in state health care reforms. *Journal of Health Politics, Policy and Law, 22*(3), 721-788.

Pandey, S. K., Mussman, M. G., Moore, H. W., Folkemer, J. G., & Kaelin, J. J. (2000). An assessment of Maryland Medicaid's rare and expensive case management program. *Evaluation and the Health Professions, 23*(4), 457-479.

Rich, R. F., & White, W. D. (1996). *Health Policy, Federalism and the American States.* Washington, DC: The Urban Institute Press.

Salganik, W. M. (2001). "'No takers for ditched Medicaid enrollees' HMOs tell panel FreeState's 40,000 not cost-effective." *Baltimore Sun.* January 26.

Salganik, W. M. (2000). " 'Health care for kids lacking,' study finds administrative glitches in Medicaid blamed." *Baltimore Sun.* November 1.

Schoenman, J. A., Evans, W. N., & Schur, C. L. (1997). Primary care case management for Medicaid recipients: Evaluations of the Maryland Access to Care program. *Inquiry, 34,* 155-70.

Sparer, M. (1996). *Medicaid and the Limits of State Health Reform.* Philadelphia, PA: Temple University Press.

Sparer, M. S., & Brown, L. D. (1996). States and the health care crisis: The limits and lessons of laboratory federalism. In Rich, R. F. and White, W. D. (Eds.), *Health Policy, Federalism and the American States.* Washington, DC: The Urban Institute Press.

Stuart, M. E., & Weinreich, M. (1998). Beyond managing care: Restructuring care. *The Millbank Quarterly, 76*(2), 251-280.

Sugg, D. (2000). Medicaid care plans penalized. State finds 4 of 8 groups aiding poor fell shy of standards $233,000 in payments held despite sanctions, officials point to gains made in year. *Baltimore Sun,* July 26.

Sundquist, J. L., & Davis, D. W. (1969). *Making Federalism Work.* Washington, DC: The Brookings Institution Press.

Thompson, F. J. (2001). "Federalism and Health Care Policy: Toward Redefinition?" In R. B. Hackey and D. A. Rochefort (Eds.), *The New Politics of State Health Policy.* Lawrence, KS: University Press of Kansas.

Thompson, F. J. (1998). The faces of devolution. In F. J. Thompson and J. J. DiIulio (Eds.), *Medicaid and Devolution: A View from the States.* Washington, DC: Brookings Institution Press.

Wasserman, M. P. (1997). Plan for long-term managed care in Maryland. (Available at *http://www.umbc.edu/chpdm/secpl197.htm*; Access Date: June 2001.)

Weiner, J. P., Tucker, A. M., Collins, A. M., Fakhraei, H., Liebermann, R., Abrams, C., Trapnell, G. R., & Folkmer, J. G. (1998). The development of risk-adjusted capitation payment system for Medicaid MCOs: The Maryland model. *Journal of Ambulatory Care Management, 21*(4), 29-52.

Wheeler, T. B. (1999). "Maryland paid MCOs millions too much." *Baltimore Sun.* February 10.

Yin, R. K. (1994). *Case Study Research: Design and Methods,* (2nd Ed.). Beverly Hills, CA: Sage.

Naturally Occurring Retirement Community-Supportive Service Program: An Example of Devolution

Patricia P. Pine, PhD

Director, New York State Office for the Aging

Vanderlyn R. Pine, PhD

Professor Emeritus, State University of New York at New Paltz

SUMMARY. Devolution is defined as the transfer of power or authority from a central government to a local government. This article addresses federal policies on housing for the elderly and the devolution of funding for federal senior housing and describes two aspects of devolution of federal housing policy for the elderly. One, it points out the decreasing interest in senior housing by federal authorities as indicated by the decreased amount of funds allocated for this purpose. Two, it emphasizes the need for supportive, assistive services for residents of senior housing and how federal funds have not addressed this need adequately or sufficiently. As a consequence, there have emerged Naturally Occurring Retirement Communities (NORCs) in New York State, a housing arrangement that provides supportive and health services to all eligible residents. The article concludes with a discussion of policy implications and the need for additional research before replicating this model. *[Article copies available for a fee from The Haworth Document Delivery Service: 1-800-HAWORTH. E-mail address: <getinfo@haworthpressinc.com> Website: <http://www.HaworthPress.com> © 2002 by The Haworth Press, Inc. All rights reserved.]*

[Haworth co-indexing entry note]: "Naturally Occurring Retirement Community-Supportive Service Program: An Example of Devolution." Pine, Patricia P., and Vanderlyn R. Pine. Co-published simultaneously in *Journal of Aging & Social Policy* (The Haworth Press, Inc.) Vol. 14, No. 3/4, 2002, pp. 181-193; and: *Devolution and Aging Policy* (ed: Francis G. Caro, and Robert Morris) The Haworth Press, Inc., 2002, pp. 181-193. Single or multiple copies of this article are available for a fee from The Haworth Document Delivery Service [1-800-HAWORTH, 9:00 a.m. - 5:00 p.m. (EST). E-mail address: getinfo@haworthpressinc.com].

10.1300/J031v14n03_10

KEYWORDS. Senior housing, affordable housing, care management, aging in place

INTRODUCTION

It has long been recognized that the basic necessities of housing and shelter for older people may be provided through alternative socio-cultural approaches. For example, in most agrarian societies, housing emerged from an extended family network, with older people remaining with younger relatives until death. Alternatively, in many feudal societies, communal cooperative living arrangements for the older and very old were typical. In some industrial societies, the old lived with their nuclear family members until they died. Finally, in certain post-industrial societies, institutional housing has become common. In the United States, there have been examples of all these approaches.

Since the early 20th century in the United States, there has been an increasing trend of older people living alone independently rather than in institutions or with either extended or nuclear families. In fact, census data point out that in 1960 about one-fifth of the elderly lived alone. By 1995, nearly one-third lived alone. Many of them require assistance from others to continue to live alone. Moreover, supportive services for independent elderly people living in the community have been provided by federal funds under the Older Americans Act since 1965. These services, including transportation to medical appointments and shopping, nutrition, counseling, group services, health prevention and health screening services, and others, are offered to people age 60 and older who are eligible, who have access, and who will pay the suggested contribution. In many cases, however, there are waiting lists of elderly people who do not live in areas where they are accessible or convenient to these services.

This paper addresses federal policies on housing for the elderly and the devolution of funding for federal senior housing. Devolution is defined as the transfer of power or authority from a central government to a local government. This paper will describe two aspects of devolution of federal housing policy for the elderly: (1) the decreasing interest in senior housing by federal authorities as indicated by the decreased amount of funds allocated for this purpose, and (2) the need for supportive, assistive services for residents of senior housing and how federal funds have not addressed this need adequately. As a consequence, there has been an emergence of Naturally Occurring Retirement Communities

(NORCs) in New York State. Under the auspices of private, not-for-profit, and subsequently, state funds, NORCs' developments provide supportive and health services to all eligible residents within existing housing. Finally, the paper presents the statistics of services provided by New York State NORCs.

THE THREE "As" OF SENIOR HOUSING

In the late 20th century, most older people have preferred to "age in place," with the support of in-home assistance and services. Even if they had moved to other housing arrangements in their earlier older years (e.g., in their 70s), older people still tend to remain in place until a critical need for institutional living arises. They cope with decline with the assistance of family, friends, and community services for as long as possible.

Two factors of housing help explain the growing trend of older people wanting to live independently. One factor is the appeal of privacy. If they can afford it, people prefer not to share living space with someone other than a spouse. In the last half of the 20th century, adults of all ages purchased and expected personal privacy in their living arrangements.

A second factor is the appeal of autonomy versus the loss of personal control over daily activities. Living independently provides autonomy, and the loss of control often accentuates both mental and physical deterioration.

To maintain a desirable level of privacy and a suitable degree of control, older people consider the three "As" of senior housing to be very important. One is *affordability*. There are many housing expenses and responsibilities that older people either cannot or do not want to continue. Some of these are major housing-related concerns, including home upkeep, failing health, and loss of independence. When incomes remain fixed or do not increase to meet inflation and market increases, the elderly are faced with the problem of affording the types of housing they want. If they are homeowners, the actual expenses for home maintenance often exceed what the owners can afford. In the last decade, 87% of elderly homeowners had mortgage-free homes, but many had older houses in need of repairs. Elders' physical abilities may have declined so that they can no longer perform previously conducted chores, and nearly 30% of their incomes were spent on housing costs. Thus, affordability is a major component of senior housing. Policies to address affordability include low-income public housing, subsidized rent, and some home maintenance/weatherization programs for household rehabilitation.

The second aspect is *availability*. Although it is estimated that over 300,000 publicly sponsored senior housing projects have been constructed over the past 40 years and nearly 45% of all public housing is occupied by the elderly, there is still an insufficient number of units to meet the demand. As the aging population continues to grow, the need for additional housing will continue. Thus, another problem of senior housing is availability of sufficient units.

The third aspect is *accessibility*. As people age, the need for accessible accommodations in their housing increases. Senior housing often includes elevators, walk-in showers, and other features associated with age-related disabilities. Most housing units constructed for senior citizens have been independent apartments or units. As the population ages, there has been an increasing demand for housing with supportive services such as meals, cleaning, laundry, transportation, and shopping. Assisted Living, Continuing Care Retirement Centers, and other models are developing rapidly across the country. Waiting lists are common, especially for affordable new developments. During the first few decades of the 21st century, there will be a continuing need for accessible senior housing.

THE HISTORY OF FEDERAL SENIOR CITIZEN
PUBLIC HOUSING

Historically, federal public housing for older people generally has addressed two social conditions: the increased demand for housing and the increasing costs of institutionalized housing (nursing homes). The number of older people is expected to increase dramatically over the next 20 to 30 years. Providing adequate housing for this increasing population will undoubtedly require federal assistance. Lower cost for or more cost-effective alternatives to nursing homes are encouraged.

In the first half of the 20th century, federal housing policy for the elderly generally was included in policies for other age groups. Policymakers first noted the needs of the elderly in the 1930s. Housing policy and initiatives began to affect the lives of the elderly and all Americans during the Economic Depression of the 1930s. Working families of all ages were affected by the difficult economic times, and the number of homeless people increased. Senior citizens were occupying substandard housing at a slightly higher rate than other households (Fisher, 1959).

The U.S. Housing Act of 1937 was passed to alleviate the housing shortage and related housing financial difficulties. It established mechanisms to assist homeowners and those constructing homes. It assisted renters by offering public subsidies for housing and the establishment of Public Housing Authorities. However, families were targeted for the subsidies, and single residents were not eligible until 1956. This factor prohibited many senior citizens, particularly widows, from being able to avail themselves of this benefit.

Private builders opposed and argued that publicly supported housing was another step toward socialism (Mason, 1982). The mission of the U.S. Housing Act often was distorted because, immediately upon enactment, the commissioner of housing spoke of the mission of the act as to "provide good homes and healthful living conditions for low income families," while supporters of this act justified its value for work relief and for slum clearance (Fisher, 1959). Both the confusion of the mission and private builders' resistance negatively affected the funding for this important housing program over the next several decades.

After World War II, the U.S. Housing Act of 1949 authorized the construction of 810,000 new housing units in six years. Support was rallied for housing for the elderly, as well as support for those with large families and for veterans (Fisher, 1959). Furthermore, managers and neighborhoods more readily accepted units rented to the elderly in an effort to avoid renting to single and unwed mothers (Meyerson, Terrett, & Wheaton, 1962).

Section 202 of the U.S. Housing Act of 1959 provided direct loans to non-profit and limited-profit sponsors, consumer cooperatives, and public agencies to construct or rehabilitate rental or cooperative housing for senior citizens and the handicapped (Ehrlich, 1976). Section 202 was designed to provide housing for the independent elderly, offering affordability, but did not provide supportive services needed for accessibility. The residents were expected to move to other accommodations, such as nursing homes, when the need arose. The Farmers' Home Administration's Section 515 program established a direct loan program for rural housing that has provided for many rural housing units for the elderly.

During the last 20 twenty years of the 20th century, federal funds for public housing and especially for senior citizen housing decreased, and any funds that were appropriated quickly had waiting lists of projects to be developed as the developers identified the need for more projects. Thus, availability of affordable senior housing was limited, and accessible housing was not acknowledged.

Because these needs were not addressed adequately, an innovative model was developed to assist the elderly who desired to "age in place." A new solution was posed. Naturally Occurring Retirement Communities (NORCs), residential housing complexes such as an apartment building or buildings, a housing development, or a housing cooperative, which is home to many older people, were developed. They were funded under the auspices of private, not-for-profit, and subsequently, state funds. People moved into the apartments as young adults, and the retirement function occurred naturally by the process of aging.

As people age, there is more integration between their housing and their health care (Pynoos & Leibig, 1995). Access to supportive health services becomes more important, and providing services on-site at the housing project becomes desirable. The Naturally Occurring Retirement Communities employ the services of housing management or local agencies to provide services under contract for all eligible residents.

Although NORCs do not substitute for new construction of senior housing, they have filled the gaps of two problems of senior housing: accessibility and affordability (and in many cases, availability). Without supportive services, many residents would need to move to higher and more costly levels of care.

NEW YORK STATE NORCs

Beginning in the mid-1980s, the United Jewish Appeal-Federation in New York City sponsored a program of social and health services at a cooperative housing project. In this project, occupants owned their individual units but shared common ownership rights, mutually agreed upon obligations and responsibilities, and pooled their economic resources to support the shared housing project. This project served more than 1,000 senior citizens a year. Over the years, the United Jewish Appeal-Federation has expanded these services to other housing sites. Their model includes:

- The program at each housing cooperative reflects the needs of its elderly residents.
- The cooperative corporations pay a substantial share of the costs of the services.
- The program at each site is directed and coordinated by an experienced social work agency.

- Each program is governed by a committee representing the cooperative's management, board of directors, elderly residents, and agencies providing the services.
- Residents of each cooperative volunteer to provide many group services.
- Plans for self-sufficiency after the initial foundation grants expire are prepared in advance of need (Lanspery & Callahan, 1994).

In 1994, after years of positive demonstration projects, the New York State Legislature declared in Section 410 of the 1994 Laws of New York State to support NORCs to assure quality of life, to access a variety of necessary services that would help residents maintain their independence, and to avoid costly and unnecessary hospital stays and nursing home placements. That year, the Legislature funded 10 projects, eight in New York City and two upstate, one in Rochester and one in Troy. By 1999, 14 projects were funded, the original 10 plus four more in New York City.

The criteria for state funding are building complexes that (1) have been constructed with funds provided by any sector of government, including loans or loan subsidies, for the purpose of construction of an apartment building or housing complex for low- or moderate-income persons as defined by the U.S. Department of Housing and Urban Development (HUD); (2) are not built originally for elderly persons; (3) does not restrict admission solely to the elderly; and (4) have elderly residents occupying 50% or a minimum of 2,500 of the housing units (for the purpose of identifying eligible units, the elderly are defined as those age 60 and older who are heads of households). A 100% match to the state funds is required, but a waiver can be secured if the project serves low-income people (New York State Office for the Aging, 2000).

The Naturally Occurring Retirement Communities address the problem of the availability of senior housing. Rather than construct new publicly funded units, NORCs enable older residents to remain in the apartment where they have lived for many years. They also address the problem of affordability, because the renter remains in the apartment, not a newly constructed, expensive unit. They also address the problem of accessibility by retrofitting the unit to be accessible by the disabled, if necessary.

Support Services Provided

The Naturally Occurring Retirement Communities address the needs of older residents, especially those living alone, by providing support services, generally on site, to its residents. Services are provided under contract and are available to all who need them on request. This is in contrast to other elderly living in the community, where support services, if available, must be individually identified, tested, and purchased. In most communities, many people receive insufficient services because they cannot find, purchase, or obtain services they may require.

In the 14 NORCs in New York State, the following service statistics on Care Management services and recipients are relevant as it is the most commonly provided service (New York State Office for the Aging, 2000). Care Management offers the older person an assessment of need and coordinates the identified services required for the person to remain independent. Although not all housing projects provide all services, the following ones are available:

- Care Management
- Case Management
- Housekeeping/personal assistance/home chores/paid escort
- Home-delivered meals
- Nursing
- Physician services
- Psychiatry-group
- Psychiatry-individual
- Counseling
- Lifeline
- MD home visits
- Crisis intervention

The following list describes the characteristics of the recipients of the Care Management services:

- *Gender:* Of the 14,399 individuals who received Care Management every year for the past five years, more than 75% of the clients are female. In 1999, 80% of those receiving Care Management were women.
- *Ethnicity:* Twelve of the fourteen New York State NORCs are located in New York City. The ethnicity of those receiving Care Management services reflects the diversity of the city. Eighty (80) percent of all recipients were white; 12% were Black. Hispanic residents constituted 6% of the recipients, and 2% were Asian/Pacific Islander.
- *Age:* Most recipients were older; 83% were over age 75. Forty-three (43) percent of the recipients of Care Management were between

75 and 84 years; 39% were over age 85; and only 17% were under age 75.

- *Household Size:* Most of the recipients lived alone, in single-person households. Seventy-seven (77) percent of the Care Management recipients lived alone.
- *Activities of Daily Living:* NORCs provide services to those older people to reduce hospitalization and other institutionalization. Thirty (30) percent of the recipients have no limitations with the Activities of Daily Living (ADLs), that is, limitations with functional self-care tasks, such as bathing, eating, dressing, transferring from bed or chair, toileting, and walking. Twenty-two (22) percent have limitations with one activity. Fifteen (15) percent have limitations with two activities, and 9% have limitations with three activities. Twenty-three (23) percent of recipients have limitations with more than three activities.
- *Instrumental Activities of Daily Living:* Care Management services provide much assistance to those who are limited in the Instrumental Activities of Daily Living (IADLs), those activities of home management, such as financial management, telephoning, walking outside, shopping, meal preparation, and safety procedures. Forty-four (44) percent of all managed care recipients have limitations with IADLs. Sixteen (16) percent have limitations with two IADLs and similarly with three activities. Eleven (11) percent have limitations with one IADL, and thirteen (13) percent have no limitations.

Group services also are provided by NORCs. The following services are offered:

- Education/recreation
- Health education and screening
- Support groups, e.g., caregiver
- Congregate meals
- Health promotion/testing
- Exercise program
- Adult day program
- Mental health awareness

Over 473,000 residents participated in the education and recreation programs. Nearly 350,000 residents utilized the support groups, although most groups have only 10 to 13 members regularly, on average. One housing project offers 294 different support groups, all with about 13 members. Others offer only one group.

Other frequently used services provided by the residents are information and referral, outreach, transportation, volunteerism, senior center visits, and shopping.

NORCs have made a substantial contribution to housing needs with support services for some elderly. Although data are not available to compare demographically the residents of NORC housing with those in other senior housing programs, such as Section 202 housing, it can be predicted that the age, gender, and household size would be similar. Providing services through NORCs' coordinated care management model probably offers more readily accessible and appropriate services. Those same services procured through the more common method of individual piece-by-piece procurement generally are not so accessible, available, and possibly not appropriate. In fact, for many service providers, funded by community or public funds, there are insufficient funds to serve all individuals in need. Thus, if the residents of Section 202 or other housing projects requested services from the available community-based providers, including the local area agency on aging, the services undoubtedly would not be available. Therefore, the organized clustered services provided by a NORC appear to be more cost-effective as well as care-effective for the residents.

POLICY IMPLICATIONS

There are major policy implications when one seeks to evaluate the value of NORCs compared to other housing programs, such as Section 202 housing. NORCs seem to work best in circumstances in which the residents have long-standing experience with cooperative activities. Specifically, people who have lived in condominium-type housing with a well-established system of governance and racial or ethnic congruence appear to adjust better to the NORC environment than others might. The importance of racially or ethnically congruent occupants and the accompanying tendency for segregationist-like exclusion is a matter that deserves further research and investigation because, while the two values have powerful benefits, they also raise many attendant policy issues in the domains of equality and equal access. Unfortunately, government policy assumes that everyday elderly (and not so elderly) people will abide by equal rights legislation, whereas just the opposite might be the case, especially in striving for harmonious communal housing arrangements.

Another major policy issue involves the legislated requirements for housing assistance. Just because someone lives in an eligible low-income complex, it raises the ecological fallacy conundrum in real life. Some of the long-time residents of a low-income project are no longer themselves what would qualify as "low" income because of inheritance, consolidation of their personal assets, or recently acquired wealth. How, then, do administrators judge whether someone living in an eligible project is personally eligible, given his or her current changed status? In truth, they probably do not. The issue, therefore, becomes one of evaluating the efficacy and efficiency of a program as it relates to actual people rather than to abstract goals. Once again, the research called for is far beyond the scope of this paper, but to judge accurately the relative comparability of NORCs versus Section 202s, that research must be done.

Another policy issue that arises involves the etiology of program devolution. It is reminiscent of the age-old question, "Which came first, the chicken or the egg?" The "transfer of authority" is really a misnomer because most of the recent federal legislation about housing for the elderly was to cut back support and not to transfer anything. This practice may reflect conceptual programmatic devolution; however, responses to the cutbacks evolved from elderly people themselves, the non-profit groups that saw a need, and the creative energies of those who thought, "there must be a better way." It then involved the evolution of new or refashioned ideas among communal living initiatives. The policy rub, of course, is should any level of government try to design a devolution model or should there be a model of government openness in responding to new programs that arise relatively spontaneously? Units of government typically are slow to respond to new challenges, but with the recent history of large-scale cutbacks, well-documented research on the value of the openness model is sorely needed, especially in the area of housing for the elderly.

CONCLUSION

Over the past 80 years, federal housing policy has focused primarily on housing construction and the financing of buildings. Over the past two decades, it has become evident that senior citizens need more than a physical structure to remain independent. They also need a wide range of support services for accessibility. Since 1990, federal budgets have included funds for support services in federally funded projects, but those funds have not been sufficient to meet the demand. Thus, availability and accessibility have been limited.

The decreased priority of federal housing policy has devolved to local programs. New York State's Naturally Occurring Retirement Communities have filled a need for affordable supportive housing that has been unmet by federal housing programs. The state-funded programs are providing accessible supportive housing for urban New Yorkers. The projects and similar creative approaches can be replicated in other communities in New York and in other states where older residents live in close proximity to each other, whether in apartment complexes, mobile home parks, or neighborhoods.

In New York State, NORCs offer needed services and have reduced or deterred the entry into nursing homes and hospitals. The costs are reasonable, which makes the housing affordable and accessible. Because the individual older person already resides in the apartment, the housing is *de facto* available.

As funding has not kept pace with the demand, through devolution from the federal government, NORCs have emerged. With the increasing number of older people expected in the next 10 to 15 years, Naturally Occurring Retirement Communities appear to be a viable option for states and communities for affordable, accessible, and available housing of senior citizens.

Although the early evidence is encouraging, more research must be conducted and concluded before Naturally Occurring Retirement Communities can be considered a superior method of providing housing and support services to the elderly. Demographic comparisons of individual needs and characteristics must be evaluated, as well as the types and costs of services provided. However, with the aging of the baby boomers, NORCs represent a method by which elders can remain in their own homes while receiving services necessary to live independently and perhaps to meet their individual expectations. The ultimate devolution-related issue is likely to be which levels or units of government, the public non-profit sector, the private sector, or some combination, will address the problem in the 21st century.

AUTHOR NOTES

Patricia P. Pine is Director of the New York State Office for the Aging. She has more than 30 years of experience in government policy, program, and service delivery in the field of aging and long-term care.

She can be contacted at the New York State Office for the Aging, 2 Empire State Plaza, Albany, NY 12223 (E-mail: pat.pine@ofa.state.ny.us).

Vanderlyn R. Pine is Professor Emeritus of Sociology at the State University of New York at New Paltz, where he was on the faculty from 1970 to 1998. He is the author or editor of eight books and dozens of articles on a wide range of sociological topics, with a special focus on social change.

He can be contacted at 16 Plattekill Avenue, New Paltz, NY 12561 (E-mail: afc@teamafc.com).

REFERENCES

Ehrlich, I. F. (1976). The politics of housing the elderly, in R. E. Mendelson and M. A. Quinn (Eds.) *The Politics of Housing: Older Urban Areas.* New York: Praeger Publishers.

Fisher, R. M. (1959). *20 Years of Public Housing.* New York: Harper & Brothers.

Lanspery, S. C., & Callahan Jr., J. J. (1994). *Naturally Occurring Retirement Communities: A Report Prepared for the Pew Charitable Trusts.* Waltham, MA: Brandeis University.

Mason, J. B. (1982). *History of Housing in the United States, 1930-1980.* Houston, TX: Gulf Publishing Company.

Meyerson, M. B., & Terrett, W. W. (1962). *Housing, People and Cities.* New York: McGraw Hill Book Company.

New York State Office for the Aging (1997). *Naturally Occurring Retirement Community Supportive Service Program, Program Report.* Albany, NY.

Pynoos, J., & Liebig, P. S. (1995). Housing policy for frail elders: Trends and implications for long-term care, in J. Pynoos and P. S. Liebig (Eds.) *Housing Frail Elders: International Policies, Perspectives, and Prospects.* Baltimore: Johns Hopkins Press.

Information Technology Issues
in an Era of Greater State Responsibilities:
Policy Concerns for Seniors

Carolyn M. Shrewsbury, PhD

Minnesota State University, Mankato

SUMMARY. Five areas of state information technology policy are of special concern to seniors and senior service providers: obtaining access; closing the digital divide; developing information management systems; creating portals; and maintaining privacy. Increasing their activities in each of these areas, states continue to vary considerably in their responsiveness to meeting the challenge of including older adults, especially those living in rural areas, with the benefits of information technology. *[Article copies available for a fee from The Haworth Document Delivery Service: 1-800-HAWORTH. E-mail address: <getinfo@haworthpressinc.com> Website: <http://www.HaworthPress.com> © 2002 by The Haworth Press, Inc. All rights reserved.]*

KEYWORDS. Internet, state government, information technology policy, aging policy

INTRODUCTION

Information technologies (IT) are transforming the ways in which we relate to our world and to each other. While policy issues about information technologies have little specific focus on older persons, many of their consequences profoundly impact seniors as well as programs and services that are targeted to them. This is especially true for those living in rural areas. Because of this impact, those interested in aging need to

[Haworth co-indexing entry note]: "Information Technology Issues in an Era of Greater State Responsibilities: Policy Concerns for Seniors." Shrewsbury, Carolyn M. Co-published simultaneously in *Journal of Aging & Social Policy* (The Haworth Press, Inc.) Vol. 14, No. 3/4, 2002, pp. 195-209; and: *Devolution and Aging Policy* (ed: Francis G. Caro, and Robert Morris) The Haworth Press, Inc., 2002, pp. 195-209. Single or multiple copies of this article are available for a fee from The Haworth Document Delivery Service [1-800-HAWORTH, 9:00 a.m. - 5:00 p.m. (EST). E-mail address: getinfo@haworthpressinc.com].

10.1300/J031v14n03_11

be generally informed on how information technology policies intersect with more traditional aging issues. The purpose of this paper is to identify those intersections, since they are being engaged by state governments.

States have become important foci for information technology policy and older persons because of the combination of the national government's devolving policy responsibilities to the states and the states' greater policy activity resulting from their own increased capacities to govern, combined with global trends that give advantage to the more flexible and diverse responses that states can provide. There is a dynamic relationship between national and state governments when it comes to policy formation and implementation. The information technology arena is one particularly in flux.

Our survey cannot be exhaustive, but it will capture some of the most pressing state issues at the interstices of aging and information technology policy in this era of dynamic intergovernmental relationships coupled with robust and innovative private and non-profit sector activity.

It is easier to examine national policy than state policy, where 50 different versions reign, especially when the policy area is in a rapid state of development. Rather than capture a snapshot of a moment in time, this paper seeks to focus on the kinds of examples that can illustrate the state policy domain. Although groups like AARP, the Spry Foundation, and the National Council on the Aging (NCOA) monitor information technology developments in the national arena, similar groups at the state and local levels have been less attentive to information technology policy. The stereotype that older persons cannot or will not use computers, send e-mail, or surf the Web is fading. However, the voice of senior interests in the states is still too rarely heard as information technology policy issues are discussed. Making some of these interests more visible is a secondary goal of this paper.

We will examine five specific information policy concerns: access, the digital divide, information management systems, state portals, and privacy. Several different intergovernmental relationships will be noted. Access, especially the ability to obtain high-speed broadband services, is an issue area once dominated by the federal government. Deregulation opened the way for state involvement, especially through public-private partnerships. The digital divide, the gap between those with and those without either access to computers and the Internet or without the skills to utilize them, presents issues where federal interest and concern may be manifest, but actual federal involvement comes primarily through grants, research, and information sharing. State and local governments are the primary public frontline actors working to narrow the digital divide, which has disadvantages for older persons, especially the rural elderly. State information management systems, computerized databases, and information processing systems demonstrate the intertwining of state and federal concerns. State portals, gateways to information and services, are areas where states can act independently and in some cases assume responsibilities, which the national government has shed. Privacy issues are a battleground between those who want the federal government to preempt the policy area and those who see the states as needing to be both individual actors in the privacy domain and as protectors against federal intrusions into privacy.

ACCESS TO INFORMATION TECHNOLOGY

Having access to information technology is the first step toward participating in its benefits. Access has several dimensions. In this section, we focus on developing the backbone infrastructure necessary to get on the information highway. While seniors in metropolitan areas may take for granted the availability of at least toll-free dial-up access to the Internet, rural elders have faced more challenges in getting online. For rural seniors (and for local service providers), this access may be even more important. When the local pharmacy has left town, searching the Internet for adaptive aids may mean not having to rely on someone who could drive you to the regional center. A medication monitoring system, either by a special device connected to the phone or by a computer connection, may allow seniors to remain in their homes instead of having to relocate to nursing homes.

Small towns have not only lost their retail base as "big box" stores in regional centers priced the small town merchant out of business; many have also lost young families to economically livelier cities. The social support networks of many areas have dwindled just as much as the economic base. As important as it may be to urban seniors, to rural seniors the Internet can offer one of the few lifelines to being able to remain in place. Access is critical for them.

The telephone is the first link in obtaining access. The Telecommunications Act of 1996 was the first major revision in telecommunications policy in over 60 years. The goal of the act is to let anyone enter any communications business. This meant a major shift from regulated monopolies to encouraging competition in the telecommunications area. Although the FCC and the national government would remain key players in telecommunications policy, one consequence of the act was to open the way for states to play more of a role.

One intersection of aging policy and telecommunications revolves around the issue of universal access. Under the old regulated system, universal access was a goal. No matter where one lived, one should have affordable access to telephone services. In the regulated system, this was facilitated by having urban areas subsidize rural ones and businesses subsidize residential service through the regulated fee structures. In the deregulated system, these subsidies would no longer exist. Many remain concerned that competition alone will not result in universal and affordable access to modern telecommunications facilities. This is especially true for obtaining broadband services in rural areas (Olufs, 1999).

Congress and the Federal Communications Commission are committed to maintaining universal service. Indeed, as a part of the 1996 Act, a joint board of federal, state, and consumer representatives was asked to make recommendations regarding universal access. In May 1997, the FCC made a decision that included the mechanisms to maintain universal access. For individuals, this universal access required traditional phone service. However, individual residential access to broadband services that would make more advanced information technologies usable was not included in this decision.

Nevertheless, the FCC has continued to be active in extending the concept of universal service. In 1999, the FCC obtained a commitment from AT&T to extend services to rural and remote areas as a condition of approval of a merger. The FCC has made similar requirements for other mergers. Under the 1996 Act, the FCC regularly reports to Congress the status of universal access goals.

One ongoing debate about how to ensure that competition leads to access, including affordable prices, involves the different ways the 1996 Act treats cable and telephone companies. In an AARP research report, Trevor R. Roycroft advocates open access for cable so that cable companies offer the same opportunities for competition among Internet access providers as must telephone companies (Roycroft, 2001).

Others who are more focused on extending service to rural areas argue that competition works against extending access to rural areas. They suggest that dropping the requirement that telephone companies allow competitors to provide Internet access to its DSL users would speed broadband availability to rural customers (Carlson, 2001). The U.S. Congress continues to discuss these issues, and Congress and the FCC remain major players in information technology policy.

As discussion about competition proceeds at the national level, states are acting to extend access, especially to ensure that broadband access is rapidly made universally available. In its 2000 legislative session, for example, North Carolina approved the creation of the Rural Internet Access Authority. One of its goals is "to provide high-speed Internet access at competitive prices . . . to all North Carolinians within the next three years" (North Carolina Rural Economic Development, 2000).

Arizona's project Topaz (Telecommunications Open Partnerships for Telecommunication Services for All Citizens of Arizona) includes a state contract with Qwest to extend services in 39 rural communities (Hull, 2000). Other public-private partnerships are envisioned.

Several states, including Minnesota, use the leverage they have in selling rights of way along interstate highways to telecommunications companies. As a condition for purchasing a right of way, the company is required to provide additional rural networks (Swope, 2000). Oregon has used similar public-private partnerships to trade fast track permitting for access (Weeldmeyer, 2000). Minnesota, as do a number of other states, also provides grants to local governments to expand high-speed access in rural areas. Often these local governments use the grants to form public-private partnerships of their own.

Governor Angus King of Maine maintains that the high penetration of telecommunications in rural Maine stems from "forward thinking businesses, the legislature passing the right kind of tax laws and a governor who keeps bugging the companies" (Peterson, 2001). The state's "vision statement" for information technology emphasizes policies that encourage the private sector to extend access to all areas of the state.

A very different approach can be seen in LaGrange, Georgia, where the city entered into a partnership with the local cable company to provide access through a custom set-top box that allows citizens to surf the net and send e-mail. By not requiring residents to have traditional computers, the city felt the system would be more accessible to all (Marcotte, 2000). Lakefield, Minnesota, is engaged in a similar project using a different technology (Sturdevant, 2000).

Thus, it can be seen that many states have identified rural access as an important state issue. While this has usually reflected concerns about economic development, the significant elderly population in rural areas could not benefit from IT without that access. The national government has not abandoned its primary role in telecommunications policy, but many states have used their opportunity to act, especially by forming public-private partnerships or using other mechanisms to facilitate private activity. Although access to the information highway is not specific to the problems faced by seniors, advocates for the aging would do well to monitor and encourage efforts to extend access, especially to rural communities.

THE DIGITAL DIVIDE

The digital divide is the gap between those who have access to information technology and those who do not, for whatever reasons. As we saw in the previous section, some problems come from lack of access to telecommunications. For example, there is a lack of access to toll-free dial up in some rural areas and to broadband services in many rural and central city areas. In this section, we focus on the other aspect of access: whether or not people have the resources and knowledge and physical ability to use existing information technologies. Many experts see these problems as the fundamental aspect of the digital divide.

The private and non-profit sectors and the federal government have focused on diminishing the digital divide. SeniorNet is one of the most successful non-profit groups actively promoting senior usage of computers and the Internet. Microsoft has been an active private sector supporter of non-profit and government efforts to expand computer usage, including older adults. At the federal government level, the Department of Commerce reports on the Digital Divide have shown a consistent gap based both on residence (rural underserved) and on age, with senior citizens underserved. (For more detail, see the chart at *http://www.ntia.doc.gov/ntiahome/fttn99/FTTN_I/Chart-I-27.html.*) However, seniors are among the fastest growing group of Internet users (1999 Internet Report by Media Metrix cited in "The Big Picture"). Efforts to increase senior usage have led to more sites of particular interest to seniors, which then increase senior usage ("Seniors and Computing"). Overall, older adults use the Internet in much the same ways that younger adults do, for example, travel, investments, e-mail, purchases, entertainment, family history, health information, current events, or looking for services (Cohen, 1998; Delmore, 2000).

States, in response to the 1996 Telecommunications Act provisions and subsequent funding of the e-rate, are undertaking to wire schools and public libraries to lessen the digital divide (Le Blanc, 2000). There is increasing recognition that, although excluded from the e-rate, wiring senior centers is a necessary part of the effort to wire central community institutions. Like schools and libraries, senior centers are a central focal point for activities and services, including education and training. Senator Ron Wyden (2000) of Oregon surveyed Oregon senior centers, finding that over half the centers did not have computers, and 70% had no Internet access. He proposed an s-rate, like the e-rate only to provide discounted Internet connections to targeted low income or rural senior centers. Former Governor Tom Ridge's administration in Pennsylvania provided grants to link up more than 90 of the state's 671 senior community centers (Gold, 2000). There are also private foundation and corporate funds being used to wire senior centers.

Some local communities have begun education and training efforts in an attempt to lessen the digital divide. Usually, these efforts are not focused on senior citizens (although some provider education classes and some senior groups have such a focus). However, West Virginia has a Seniors Technology Training Program, a partnership among West Virginia, Microsoft, and Marshall University (Underwood, 1999). Some senior Web sites provide tutorials, information, and other access information. Some Area Agencies on Aging have sponsored training.

The amount and kind of training needed to lessen the digital divide depends on the minimum information technology goal. Some maintain that the definition of universal service must expand to include the new components: (1) access to the World Wide Web, (2) an e-mail address, and (3) the capability to make one's own information available via the Web (see "Losing Ground Bit by Bit," 1998, for the advocacy view and Bonnett, 1996, for a more analytic view).

To achieve bridging of the digital divide, intergenerational projects often connect seniors and at-risk youth to combine training for seniors with mentoring for youth. One such project reported by the Rural Telecommunications Congress, the Youth Elderly Linkage Project, had at-risk high school students working with seniors to learn how to use the Internet to access more health information, other educational activities, and e-mail with family. (This and other rural projects can be accessed at *http://ruraltelecon.org/projects.asp.*)

Internet use may be especially important for frail elderly. In one study of older adults from the nursing and independent living sections of a retirement community, those who were taught to use e-mail and the Internet experienced a decrease in loneliness (White et al., 1999). Another study found that Internet use helped combat depression among nursing home residents (Noer, 1995). Wright (2000) found that the Internet provided a viable support network via chat rooms and message boards for some seniors.

Income differences may increase the digital divide as more advanced uses of IT develop. Aging-related services are increasingly focusing on ways to use Internet technologies to increase the quality of their services, lower administrative costs or provide better management information, decrease the costs of their services, and market their services (Anderson, 1998). Oatfield Estates, a residential care complex by Elite Care in a Portland, OR, suburb, is an example of a completely wired and partially automated long-term care facility (Berck, 2001). Whether or not this is the improvement in care that Elite Care believes it to be remains to be validated, either by empirical research or by the marketplace. The same could be said for the developments that are beginning to allow "smart homes" that can compensate for frailty as well as cater to the indulgent (Eisenberg, 2001). Unless state regulators intervene, it is likely that assisted living facilities catering to higher income seniors will be wired and have extensive IT use, while facilities aimed at more moderate-income persons will not.

State Regulatory agencies can play another role in addressing the digital divide. In Ohio, AARP was one of several clients represented in a negotiated settlement with Ameritech that provided for the establishment of 14 community computing centers ("Losing Ground Bit by Bit," 1998).

The national government continues to have some role in lessening the digital divide. One role of the federal government in helping rural communities with access to information technology is the provision of grants. By 1996, there were already 28 federal programs providing such grants ("Rural Development," 1996). For example, senior organizations, often in partnership with local governments, participate in the TIIAP (Telecommunications and Information Infrastructure Assistance Program) and the Department of Housing and Urban Development's Neighborhood Networks Initiative, which provides training and access to residents of HUD financed properties.

The digital divide has already lessened and it will continue to do so. However, there are some special concerns regarding the elderly. A large percentage of those not currently using the Internet and e-mail have no desire to do so. The move to smart devices that do not require specific knowledge by the user would allow senior use without the necessity of learning a new technology. However, until the time when information technology is totally transparent, states will need to continue projects that incorporate uses that are important to seniors and make it possible for them to access such uses. Further, while many seniors will be well served by moves to e-government and to Web-based services, those that will not must not be ignored. Off-line channels will need to be maintained and targeted to those who remain on the wrong side of the digital divide ("Survey Government and the Internet," 2000).

STATE AND LOCAL GOVERNMENT INFORMATION MANAGEMENT SYSTEMS

Another policy focus concerns the development of information systems within and between state and local governments and the national government. The creation of such systems might seem to be just a management tool. While they are that, they can also be part of an overall change in the way services are conceived and delivered. This is especially true for the aging area. For example, older adults may find themselves eligible for both Medicare and Medicaid. They may also receive services from a variety of different funding streams, state, local, and federal levels of government, and non-profit and for profit organizations. Providing the same information to numerous different provider groups can result in lost information. It is also onerous for the clients. Providing it once to an integrated system shared by a multitude of groups could provide safer, better care.

Thus, information management systems should actually work for the benefit of older persons even as they fulfill the management objectives of providers and governmental units. An example of this is the Robert Wood Johnson Foundation project, Medicare/Medicaid Integration Program, which is ultimately intended to make the care for seniors less burdensome for them (National Chronic Care Consortium, 2000).

Another example is New York State's Aging Network Client Based Service Management Project. This project is financed in part by a grant from the Department of Commerce to use information technology to improve service to clients and improve agency and service provider effectiveness (Dawes, 1997). Since services in many states are provided by different agencies and different units of government as well as by a large number of non-profit and proprietary firms, other states are looking at New York's experience for developing their own systems.

There are numerous state projects for data-sharing partnerships between the public sector and private and non-profit sector organizations (see National Chronic Care Consortium, 2001, for examples from the health care field). Some projects exist to integrate public payment and reporting systems with nursing homes and other provider groups. Many of these systems are part of larger state projects for automation and integration of many of their business systems (Cats-Baril & Thompson,

1995). Other systems are aimed at detecting fraud in programs like Medicaid. For example, a Texas project allows checking to see if the same person was claimed to be treated on the same day by a doctor, hospital, and nursing home (Kittower, 1999).

Other policy issues for the aging community involve the provision of public information. One concern is how readily and in what form information like citations for nursing homes or disciplinary actions of medical practitioners should be provided. A Missouri project allows users to request background information on caregivers for children, the elderly, or the ill (*http://www.gov.state.mo.us/background/*). There is considerable debate about how much of the information collected by states should be readily available to the public and in what forms that information should be provided. State units on aging and senior organizations could cooperate to be effective advocates for maximizing public information.

In an information age, good data are essential for effective operation. Although elder services are being merged and are becoming parts of large conglomerates, many, especially in rural areas, remain small, underfunded, and dependent on volunteers, Both the national government, through reporting requirements for the Older Americans Act, and state governments have been working to improve the information reporting systems. The dilemma for these small organizations is to enhance their management systems without overly increasing their administrative overhead and losing the benefits of the flexibility inherent in their traditional operations. State governments may have a role to play in supporting these efforts.

STATE PORTALS

As information has becomes a major currency, governments find their roles shifting. Information provision has always been an important governmental function, but the variety of information that many feel government should make available is expanding. Further, the Internet has made it possible for government to provide information services 24 hours a day, seven days a week. It allows information to be available when people need it or want it. State portals should allow people actually to locate that information by providing a simple entry point.

The effectiveness of government services may then depend on how well government can anticipate what information citizens will want or need. Most state units on aging provide basic Web sites that describe their services and programs. Some provide information on current topics, for example, what to do if your HMO is terminated (Arizona) or hurricane preparation (Florida) or the dangers of summer heat (New York). Many provide basic agency information, including mission statements, plans, and staff. Most provide e-mail access to the agency, although phone access is featured most prominently on many sites. Most have links to other agencies or sites. Some have basic demographic, legal, and other educational information. A few have agency publications online. A very few have extensive lists of providers, or search engines to find providers, housing, or other aging services in one's area. Fewer yet provide downloadable forms or automatic form submission, and even fewer have any online assessment tools. A few mention state legislation related to aging issues and services. Some keep a calendar of upcoming events. None has clearly focused on each of the possible client groups (seniors, families, and caretakers), providers, provider employees, local governments, and advocates.

States continue to upgrade their portals. Virginia is one of several states that allow the public to look up licensing information on health professionals. Indiana includes report cards on nursing homes in the state so consumers can compare the quality of the facilities. Oregon allows consumers to check on whether caregivers have passed a background check and are approved by the state. Florida is linking health-related information together on one site for easy consumer access.

A good portal is especially important to rural elderly. The Administration on Aging maintains a page of resources for Web development (*http://www.aoa.dhhs.gov/aoa/pages/guidrev.html*). Only a small number of states have relatively comprehensive sites; Florida, Hawaii, and New York are among those that stand out.

PRIVACY

In May 2000, the FCC released a report, *Privacy Online: Fair Information Practices in the Electronic Marketplace*, which sought additional regulatory authority to safeguard the privacy of Web users. While some argue for preemption of privacy issues by the federal government (see, for example, Peterson, 2001), states are actively involved in privacy issues. The state of Michigan, for example, filed a lawsuit against the Department of Health and Human Services to overturn a federal law that forces the state to collect Social Security numbers whenever anyone applies for a driver's or other license (Martin, 2001).

All levels of government are struggling with what information to make available over the Internet. Seniors might share some of the concerns of police officers and other public employees about ready availability of detailed Geographic Information Systems that might compromise their safety if names are linked to such items as property information and tax records ("GIS and the Privacy Puzzle," 1999). Elderly are also special targets of scams, and the Internet broadens their vulnerability, especially as government makes information about citizens readily available.

Assuring the security of communications is an important aspect of privacy. A number of states are looking at a public key infrastructure technology that would allow citizens and businesses to know that their transactions with government, and, in some states private transactions, are secure (Towns, 2001). Almost every state has passed or is considering digital signature legislation.

A burgeoning issue related to privacy is the use of "granny cams," video-monitoring equipment, in nursing homes. Families may install these devices to have virtual visits with the resident, or to monitor their care. Advocates in some states are seeking legislation that regulates the uses of granny cams, including issues of who could consent to their use and how privacy would be protected (Edwards, 2000; Burgess, 2000).

Privacy is important to everyone. The extensive use that older persons make of health facilities and government services, their vulnerability to fraud, and the frailty of some make issues of privacy raised by the advances in information technology a necessary focus for aging advocates.

CONCLUSIONS

One of the problems with developing information technology policies encompassing senior needs and concerns is that both policies and needs are so diverse. It is hard to see the big picture. For example, regulating legal software on the Internet is an issue for many states (Newcombe, 1999). For seniors, this is especially important for estate planning, for medical directives, and for powers of attorney. But it is a narrow issue, far removed from concerns about job training for seniors who want to work but need some updating on computer technology.

We have addressed five general topics where aging issues intersect with information technology policy: access, the digital divide, information management systems, state portals, and privacy. In each of these we see the states taking increasingly active roles. As a result, around the country, there are widely varying activities in these areas. Some governors have made major commitments to improving access to information technology for older adults as well as other citizens. Some state units on aging have been proactive in developing a portal that can be used effectively by older adults and those who care for them. The downside, of course, of state rather than national action is that although some states may forge ahead with innovative policy solutions, others will remain behind. Where an elder lives has a major bearing on the access to and usefulness of information technology.

Development of integrated policy perspectives takes extensive public discussion. At this point, increasing discussion about seniors and information technology may be the necessary precursor to information technology activity in some states and to the development of a full-blown integrated policy perspective. Until the broader policy perspective can be discussed, specific questions may need to be asked over and over. For example, why are assisted living facilities being built without each unit being wired for high-speed access to the Internet? How can Sally be more regularly involved in her mother's care management even when she is 2000 miles away? Why cannot a client fill out just one form with all his/her pertinent information rather than forms for each different agency serving the client? Why cannot the senior residing in the small town have the same access to a virtual support group as her/his suburban cousin? Why does not the state technology plan consider goals that encompass older citizens?

As states involve themselves more and more in information technology issues, senior interests must be represented in policy discussions. Careful evaluation of information technology uses will help separate the hype surrounding IT from the uses that will truly enrich the quality of life of elders, contribute to the care of frail elderly as well as increase the productivity of government and non-profit agencies working with or serving older persons.

AUTHOR NOTES

Carolyn M. Shrewsbury is Professor of Political Science at Minnesota State University, Mankato.

Dr. Shrewsbury can be contacted at 109 Morris Hall, Minnesota State University, Mankato, MN 56001 (E-mail: cbury@mnsu.edu).

REFERENCES

Anderson, R. (1998). Internet comes to home care. *Caring, 17*(6), 26-8.

Berck, J. (2001, April 5). The wired retirement home. *New York Times.*

Bonnett, T. W. (1996) *Telewars in the States: Telecommunications Issues in a New Era of Competition.* Washington, DC: Council of Governors Policy Advisors.

Burgess, K. L. (2000). Grannycams raise privacy, legal issues. *Provider, 26*(4), 43-4.

Carlson, C. (2001, April 30). Taking net services rural. *eWeek, 18,* 18.

Cats-Baril, W., & Thompson, R. (1995). Managing information technology projects in the public sector. *Public Administration Review, 55*(6), 559-566.

Cohen, S. (1998). *1998 SeniorNet Study.* New York: Charles Schwab and Company.

Dawes, S. E. A. (1997, June). Tying a sensible knot: Best practices in state-local information systems. *http://www.ctg.albany.edu/resources/pdfrpwp/iis1.pdf.* Center for Technology in Government.

Delmore, S. (2000). Cybersocial seniors. *Contemporary Long Term Care, 23*(11), 38.

Edwards, D. J. (2000). All eyes are on granny cams. *Nursing Homes Long-Term Care Management, 49*(11), 27-30.

Eisenberg, A. (2001, April 5). A 'smart' home to avoid the nursing home. *New York Times.*

Finn, J. (1997). Aging and information technology. *Generations, XXI*(3).

GIS and the Privacy Puzzle. (1999, December). *Governing,* 60-1.

Gold, B. (2000). Busy Internet month in Pennsylvania. Government technology, *http://www.govtech.net/news/news.phtml?docid=2000.02.18-1015000000000179.*

Hull, J. D. (2000, December 21). New economy to boost development services in rural Arizona. Press release from the office of Jane Dee Hull, Governor, State of Arizona.

Kittower, D. (1999, October). Scale models. *Governing,* 46-52.

Le Blanc, J. (2000). Digital divide: Evolving awareness and evolving solutions. *The Digital Beat, 2*(23), *www.benton.org/DigitalBeat/.*

Losing Ground Bit by Bit: Low-Income Communities in the Information Age. (1998, July). *www.benton.org/Library/low-income/:.*

Marcotte, J. (2000). Everybody, Internet. *Government Technology,* 48-9.

Martin, W. E. (2001). By the numbers. *Government Technology,* 68-70.

National Chronic Care Consortium. (2001). *Integrating Information: Selected Issues.* Maryland: University of Maryland Center on Aging. (MMIP Technical Assistance Paper No 10 of the Robert Wood Johnson Foundation Medicare/Medicaid Integration Program).

Newcombe, P. (1999, December). Lassoing legal software. *Government Technology,* 32-34.

Noer, M. (1995). Senior cybernauts: Internet access benefits for elderly. *Forbes, 156*(7), 240-2.

North Carolina Rural Economic Development Center. (2000). Rural Internet Access Authority. Raleigh, NC, also at *http://www.ncruralcenter.org/internet/:* NC Rural Economic Development Center.

Olufs III, D. W. (1999). *The Making of Telecommunications Policy.* Boulder: Lynne Reiner.

Peterson, S. (2001, January). Gov. King of Maine. *Government Technology,* 18-22, 69.

Roycroft, T. R. (2001). *Tangled Web: The Internet and Broadband Open Access Policy.* Washington, DC: AARP Public Policy Institute.

Rural Development Steps Towards Realizing the Potential of Telecommunications. (1996, June). Technologies Report to the Committee on Agriculture, Nutrition, and Forestry, U.S. Senate. Washington, DC: GAO. (RXED-96-155).

Rural Telecommunications Congress. Rural Telecommunications Projects [Data File]: *http://206.168.125.58/projects.asp.*

Seniors and Computing. (no date). Accessed on July 5, 2000, on the Access America for Seniors Web site at *http://www.seniors.gov/computers.htm.*

Sturdevant, L. (May 25, 2000). Town aims to use telecommunications for rural makeover. *Star Tribune*, p. 25.

Survey Government and the Internet Haves and Have Nots. (2000, June 24). *The Economist, http://www.economist.com/editorial/freeforall/20000624/su2688.htl.*

Swope, C. (2000, January). Lining up telecom for rural areas. *Governing*, 55.

Towns, S. (2001, May). Security blanket public key infrastructure unlocks e-government potential. *Government Technology*, 26-33, 72.

Underwood, C. (1999, July 23). Bridging the digital divide in rural America for older adults. Press release from *AgeLight*.

Weeldmeyer, C. (2000, January). Building broadband to rural America. *Government Technology*.

White, H., McConnell, E., Clipp, E., Bynum, L., Teague, C., Mavas, L., Craven, S., & Halbrecht, H. (1999). Surfing the Net in later life: A review of the literature and pilot study of computer use and quality of life. *Journal of Applied Gerontology, 18*(3), 358-378.

Wright, K. (2000). Computer-mediated social support, older adults and coping. *Journal of Communication, 50*(3), 100-118.

Wyden, R. (2000, June 1). Oregon seniors and the digital divide: A survey of senior centers' Internet access in the new millennium, *Agelight. http://www.agelight. org/news/oregonsuvey.htm:.*

PRIVATE SECTOR INITIATIVES

A Consumer Cooperative Association Specializing in Services for the Elderly

Masato Oka, MSc

Yokohama City University, Yokohama, Japan

SUMMARY. Over the past 10 years, a Japanese cooperative association named Fukushi Club Seikyo (FCS) has developed a unique, non-profit business specializing in services for the elderly. It aims to promote a reciprocal support system among neighborhood community members. FCS has successively organized its active members, mainly homemakers, into workers' collectives and successfully provided various life support services at a very small charge. Their human-touch service appears in sharp contrast to bureaucratic public services and profit-making private services. The civil initiative presented by FCS suggests a potential for a community-based social service system that may guarantee quality services without raising taxes and premiums for social insurance. *[Article copies available for a fee from The Haworth Document Delivery Service: 1-800-HAWORTH. E-mail address: <getinfo@haworthpressinc.com> Website: <http://www.HaworthPress.com> © 2002 by The Haworth Press, Inc. All rights reserved.]*

[Haworth co-indexing entry note]: "A Consumer Cooperative Association Specializing in Services for the Elderly." Oka, Masato. Co-published simultaneously in *Journal of Aging & Social Policy* (The Haworth Press, Inc.) Vol. 14, No. 3/4, 2002, pp. 211-231; and: *Devolution and Aging Policy* (ed: Francis G. Caro, and Robert Morris) The Haworth Press, Inc., 2002, pp. 211-231. Single or multiple copies of this article are available for a fee from The Haworth Document Delivery Service [1-800-HAWORTH, 9:00 a.m. - 5:00 p.m. (EST). E-mail address: getinfo@haworthpressinc.com].

10.1300/J031v14n03_12

KEYWORDS. Consumer cooperative association, workers' collective, NPO, welfare-mix, community-based social service, Japan

INTRODUCTION

In Japan, the conventional welfare state system has been in trouble as the national finance has come to a crisis point under prolonged recession and rapid population aging. Building a new optimal welfare mix system is one of the major challenges facing Japan in the early 21st century and will require the cooperation of national and local governments, private enterprises, non-profit organizations, individuals, and families. Against this background, a consumer cooperative association named the Seikatsu Club Seikyo Kanagawa (Life Club Cooperative Association in Kanagawa Prefecture established in 1971, henceforth SCSK) and its group organizations have developed innovative activities. SCSK aims to establish a total life support system in the neighborhood community through active participation of citizens. A previous article already outlined the activities of the SCSK group with special reference to a unique nursing home named the Rapport Fujisawa (Oka, 2000a).

In 1989, SCSK's sister cooperative association, called the "Fukushi Club Seikyo" (Welfare Club Cooperative Association, henceforth FCS), was inaugurated. It aimed at responding to the needs of older persons based on the spirit of mutual support among neighborhood community members. FCS was the first experiment in the consumer cooperative movement of Japan.

Unique cooperative associations called "workers' collectives" have played an important role in the activities of the FCS. The collectives not only make contracts with the FCS to provide various services for the elderly, they also participate in the decision making process of FCS.

This article examines the activities of the FCS group that may suggest a model of non-profit organizations serving the elderly in a welfare community supported by the active participation of citizens.

HISTORY AND BACKGROUND

In the early 1980s, public opinion was highly critical on the failure of public social services for older persons. The so-called social hospitalization and lonely death of the frail elderly symbolized it. The mass media attacked the government for failing to provide necessary facilities and in-home care support services. At the same time, the Japanese socioeconomic structure was changing rapidly. The number of nuclear families was increasing and the proportion of housewives engaging in part-time jobs had reached around 50%. This meant that the traditional caregiving role of the family was in danger of breaking down.

Preparation for the FCS project started in the mid-1980s as a result of the foresight of Mr. Katsumi Yokota, the founder of SCSK. He agreed with the criticism of poor performance leveled against the Japanese welfare state. At the same time, his view was that people wanted neither a heavy burden and high social security premiums nor large expenditure for buying private service. To him it seemed that older people wanted to retain their lives in the community where they lived. Considering such crucial needs, he felt that SCSK should develop a mutual support system that would meet the challenge of the aging society (interview with Mr. K. Yokota, 2001).

Yokota also recognized that the needs of SCSK members were changing. The average age of the first generation of SCSK members was approaching 50, and the second generation (baby boomers) was about 40. They had joined SCSK to obtain safe foods for their children. However, this need declined after the child-raising period. Members who had lost their initial motivation for the joint bulk purchase of daily goods were going to retire gradually from SCSK. Moreover, a considerable increase of working women in the early 1980s led to a decline in the recruitment of new members. To deal with this situation, it was necessary for SCSK to start a new business that would meet the challenge caused by changing lifestyles of the membership (interview with Mr. K. Yokota, 2001).

The business plan made in 1987 included three pillars. The first was a home delivery service of daily goods for the households of frail elderly and relevant persons who could not join the joint purchase activities of SCSK. The second was a home help service and related daily life support service for the elderly such as rental service of care instruments. The third was a housing service by the construction of a care home and other relevant facilities responding to the housing needs of the elderly. In developing this plan, the leaders expected the members to organize workers' collectives and provide most of the actual services in order to realize the ideal of cooperative values (SCSK, 1991, pp. 266-268; Kanagawa Workers' Collective Rengo Kai, 2000, pp. 40-41).

The initial response of SCSK members was doubt about the feasibility of such an ambitious plan. However, Yokota successfully persuaded the core members to join the new activity, as "Today's caregivers should be tomorrow's care-receivers" (interviews with Mr. K. Yokota and Ms. Y. Ogawa, 2001).

The business started on an experimental basis in the northern Yokohama area in 1987 with 386 members. Two workers' collectives were formed: one for the home delivery service (22 members) and another for the home help service (26 members). In 1989, FCS obtained the legal status of an independent consumer cooperative association with a membership of 1,020. Annual sales were approximately 100 million yen (U.S. $833,000, if $1 is 120 yen). However, cost exceeded sales. This situation was gradually improved with supports from SCSK. In 1993, FCS earned a modest net surplus from the goods delivery service. Since then, FCS has shown rapid growth. As of FY 2000 ending March 31, 2001, the membership was 13,271. The annual sales of the home-delivery service were 2.7 billion yen ($22.6 million). The total amount of invested capital was 558 million yen ($4.6 million) that were reserved from rebates to each member in proportion to the amount of purchase (see Table 1).

The remaining two pillars of business have also recorded remarkable progress since FY 1994, as presented in Table 2 and explained later. As of FY 2000, the number of paid employees was only 38. There were 31 workers' collectives with a total of 1,553 members that engaged in actual service in the 21 municipalities of the Kanagawa Prefecture (FCS, 2000, pp. 8-13, 125-141; Minutes of FCS Board of Directors, 1999-2001; SCSK Movement Group, 2000, pp. 99-101; Kanagawa Workers' Collective Rengo Kai, 2000, pp. 19-39).

The current relationship between FCS and SCSK is as equal partners in the SCSK Movement Group that aims at coordinating economic, so-

TABLE 1. Progress of FCS

	FY 1989	FY 1994	FY 1999	FY 2000
Membership	1,020	6,594	12,247	13,271
Invested-capital	¥8,000 $66,700	¥176,050 $1,467,100	¥514,870 $4,290,600	¥557,900 $4,649,200
Sales of goods delivery service	¥100,000 $833,300	¥1,396,350 $11,636,300	¥2,601,260 $21,677,100	¥2,707,320 $22,561,000

Note: ¥: Japanese 1,000 Yen. $: U.S. Dollar. The assumed exchange rate: $1 = 120 Yen.
Source: Minutes of FCS Board of Directors, 2000 & 2001

cial, and political initiatives toward an alternative society based on active participation of citizens. The Group is composed of seven organizations with a total of 70,000 members. Both FCS and SCSK are consumer cooperatives. The difference between the two associations is that FCS specializes in services for the elderly and integrates the workers' collectives as a basic component of its activities, while SCSK serves all generations and relies on voluntary activities of homemakers for its joint purchase unit called "HAN" (Oka, 2000a, p. 99).

The organizational structure of FCS is explained in the next section, with detailed information on the workers' collectives. The section

TABLE 2. Development of Workers' Collectives (W.Co.) of FCS

		FY 1989	FY 1994	FY 1999	FY 2000
Home delivery service and care service ('Caretakers')	No. of W.Co. *	1	5	9	9
	Membership	22	379	622	670
	Sales	n.a.	¥99,127 ** $826,000	¥175,646 $1,464,000	¥183,808 $1,523,000
Home help and Care service ('Helpers')	No. of W.Co.	1	4	9	9
	Membership	26	213	546	570
	Sales	n.a.	¥8,914 $74,300	¥43,783 $364,900	¥112,400 $937,000
Meals-on-wheels service	No. of W.Co.	0	1	3	4
	Membership	0	15	60	82
	Sales	0	¥1,196 $10,000	¥71,059 $592,200	¥81,000 $675,000
Transportation service	No. of W.Co.	0	0	0	1
	Membership	0	0	0	12
	Sales	0	0	0	¥1,550 $12,900
Others***	No. of W.Co.	0	1	8	8
	Membership	0	4	184	219
	Sales	0	n.a.	n.a.	n.a.
Total	No. of W.Co.	2	11	29	31
	Membership	48	735	1,392	1,553
	Sales****	n.a.	¥109,237 $910,300	¥290,488 $2,420,700	¥378,758 $3,156,300

Note:
* No. of W.Co.: Number of workers' collectives organized by FCS.
** ¥: Japanese 1,000 Yen. $: U.S. Dollar. The assumed exchange rate: $1 = 120 Yen.
*** 'Others' include workers' collectives engaging in clerical and supportive services at the FCS headquarters and delivery centers.
**** 'Sales' of 'Total' is the sum except 'Others.'
Source: Minutes of FCS Board of Directors, 2000 & 2001.

"Business Performance of FCS" examines the business performance of FCS over the past 10 years. The effects on FCS caused by a public long-term care insurance system, enforced in FY 2000, are discussed in "Social Service Reform and FCS."

ORGANIZATIONAL STRUCTURE OF FCS

The current organizational structure of FCS is presented in Figure 1. Looking at the upper part of the figure, it is almost the same as the structure of ordinary consumer cooperatives. The characteristics of FCS organization are observed at the lower part of the figure and its organic relation to the upper part. The members shown at the top and the bottom of the figure are the same FCS members. They are playing various roles in the organization.

In the case of ordinary consumer cooperatives, member-customers are the masters of the organization and put daily business operations under the control of their representatives and paid employees. In the case of FCS, while the members are still the masters, unique cooperative associations called "workers' collectives" are playing a special role in the FCS organization. FCS recommends that the members organize and join workers' collectives in order to share positive roles. FCS makes a business tie-up contracts with the workers' collectives and contracts out various life support services for the frail member-customers. The workers' collectives also participate in the decision making process of FCS.

Yokota, the founder of FCS, originated this new idea for the organization of FCS. He identified the following reasons. First, he thought that the organizational nature of the workers' collective might be in tune with the genuine cooperative values of members. He took the idea from the western cooperative movement called the "producers' cooperatives," in which "the workers invest money, organize their own skills and abilities, and run a business using a self-management cooperative body system" (Yokota, 1991, p. 17). Second, he expected that workers' collectives would socialize the traditional caregiving work of women and reorganize such unpaid work into "community work" that would respond to the needs of older persons in a collective way. Third, he thought that workers' collectives would support the self-actualization of women by enabling them to manage their own work. In addition to these theoretical reasons, he wanted to utilize human resources, developed in the activities of SCSK, because the new experiment of FCS needed the experience and wisdom of homemakers (interview with Mr. K. Yokota, 2001).

During the start-up phase of FCS, there were only two workers' collectives with a membership of 48. In FY 2000, these figures increased to 31 bodies with a membership of 1,553 (see Table 2). It means that 11.7% of FCS members participated in workers' collectives. The rest were member-customers and/or care-receiving members. FCS intends to increase the ratio to 20% as a step toward realizing the ideal of mutual support among members (FCS, 2001, Minutes of the Board of Directors).

With regard to the organizational features of workers' collectives, approximately 60% of members were aged 30 to 55, and 30% were in the 56 to 65 age group. They were originally amateur groups with a few expert and qualified persons. However, recently the ratio of qualified persons such as social workers, care managers, and home helpers has been increasing as members obtain qualifications. There were no paid personnel and also no volunteers in a conventional sense as the members shared investment, management, and work in their associations. Their earnings were decided according to participating hours in the activities of the association. In some associations, small monthly allowances of less than 10 thousand yen ($83) were paid to leaders and coordinators for their additional roles. The current leaders are mainly baby boomers aged 45 to 55 with college or high school education. They are the second generation of the FCS leaders; the regeneration of the organization has been a success (Oka, 2000b, p. 38).

As shown in Figure 1, the workers' collectives are playing a major role in the management system of FCS as Yokota predicted in the mid-1980s.

The Annual Congress consisting of 120 representatives is the supreme decision making body of FCS. Most of the representatives are elected from active members of workers' collectives, since many of the FCS members are care-receivers and are unable to play major roles. The Congress elects 20 members of the Board of Directors and two auditors. The board elects one chairperson, two vice-chairpersons, and one managing director. The first chairperson was Yokota. In 1999, a woman who had considerable experience in the activities of workers' collectives succeeded him in the position. The current vice-chairpersons are also women with similar backgrounds. The managing director is a man with long service in SCSK and FCS (FCS, 2000, pp. 114-115; interviews with Ms. Tagawa and Mr. Hamada, the current leaders of FCS, 2001).

FIGURE 1. Organizational Structure of FCS

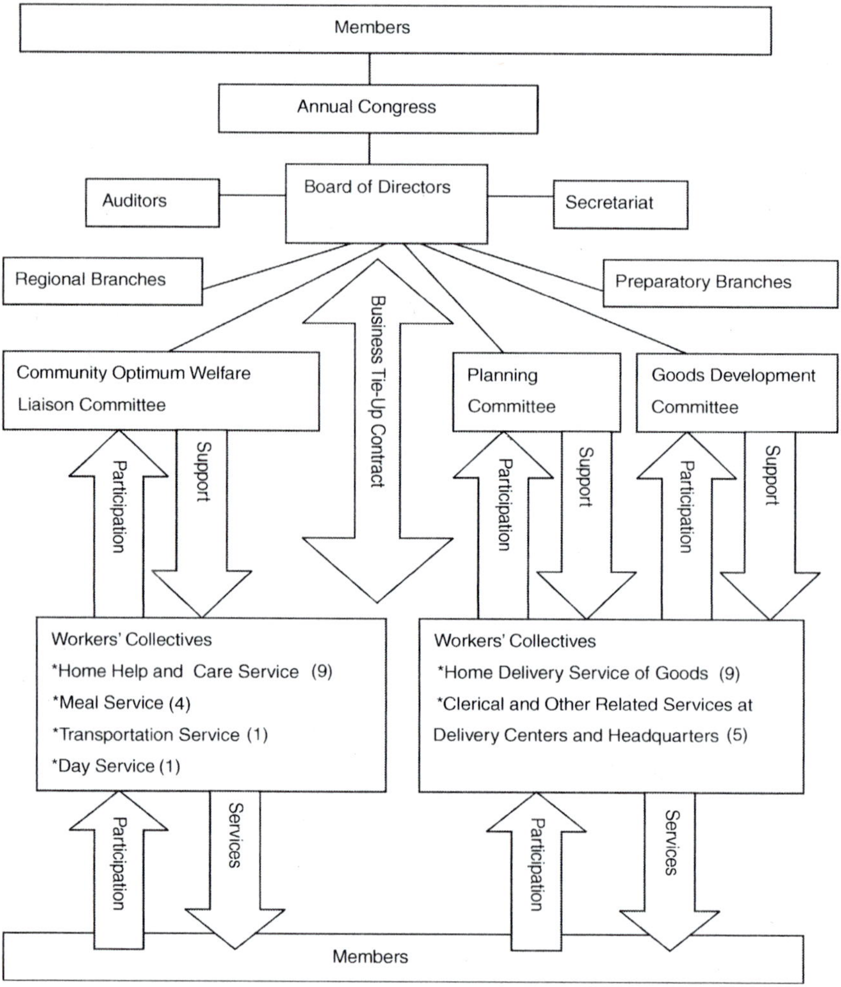

Under the Board of Directors, there are three standing committees. First, the Planning Committee has responsibility for devising the strategic plans for the home delivery service of goods. Its membership consists of the representatives of nine workers' collectives, the heads of four delivery centers, four board members, and six paid employees engaging in clerical jobs at the headquarters. Second, the Goods Development Committee has responsibility for developing new goods and improving the delivery system for the home delivery service. Its membership consists of 18 representatives of workers' collectives, two board members and two paid employees. Third, the Liaison Committee for Community Optimum Welfare has responsibility for coordinating the activities of workers' collectives engaged in the home help service, meal service, and other life support services. The key members are again the representatives of relevant workers' collectives. They exchange information, discuss the quality and price of services, and decide the strategy for further development (FCS, 2000, pp. 117-120).

The secretariat currently consists of 15 paid employees engaging in managerial and clerical jobs at the headquarters. A workers' collective was established in 1995 in order to share the duties of paid employees. In the beginning, the role of the workers' collective was limited to assistant jobs for the paid employees, but it has gradually expanded into more important managerial jobs. Another 23 paid employees are working at four delivery centers of FCS. In the delivery centers, workers' collectives with a total of 126 memberships collaborate with the paid employees. The leaders of FCS expect that more equal partnership should be developed between workers' collectives and paid employees in the near future.

FCS currently has four branches called the regional councils. Their aims are to deal with the specific issues arising in areas where membership exceeds 1,000 people. Each branch is responsible for coordinating activities of workers' collectives, devising new services, and organizing new members and workers' collectives. In the areas that have memberships of more than 700, there are currently four preparatory branches. The leaders of the workers' collectives are playing a major role in the branch activities. The division of power is the basic principle of the FCS organization (FCS, 2000, p. 123).

BUSINESS PERFORMANCE OF FCS

Home Delivery Service of Daily Goods

The basic aim of this service is to deliver safe and nutritious food and other relevant goods for healthy and successful aging. The majority of member-customers are elderly people who find shopping difficult.

The operators of this home delivery service are workers' collectives called "Sewayaki" (Caretakers). In the early days of FCS, Caretakers were recruited from among active members of SCSK. Currently, healthy members of FCS are the major source of Caretakers. Their main job is to receive goods from the delivery center of FCS and deliver them to member-customers' homes once a week. Each Caretaker is responsible for between 10 and 20 member-customers. The delivery of goods provides the opportunities for the provision of various additional services. For example, Caretakers help member-customers write order sheets of goods and put the delivered foods in the refrigerator on request. They also check on the general situation of the member-customer. If member-customers require help, they provide necessary support and information. They also introduce relevant services provided by other workers' collectives of the FCS group. Such human-touch services look very different from services provided by profit-making enterprises and bureaucratic public services.

In the initial stage, FCS was almost entirely dependent on SCSK for supplying goods. However, sometimes these were not appropriate for the particular needs of the elderly. FCS made continuous efforts to develop new goods and improve its distribution system. In FY 1993, the business recorded its first surplus of 13 million yen ($108,000) out of total sales of 1 billion yen ($8.3 million). This success gave FCS the confidence to develop further (FCS, 2000, p. 116).

The performance of the goods delivery service between FY 1994 and 2000 was remarkable. The annual sales and member-customers doubled, and the total invested capital trebled (see Table 1).

In the same period, the number of Caretakers increased from five bodies with a membership of 379 to nine bodies with a membership of 670. Their total annual sales increased 86% from 99 million yen ($826,000) to 184 million yen ($1.5 million), as shown in Table 2. Recently, Caretakers have enlarged their activities and have taken on jobs at the delivery centers of FCS, such as picking, packing, shipping, bookkeeping, which were formerly the jobs of paid employees of FCS. On average, each member of the Caretakers worked about 300 hours and earned 264,000 yen ($2,200) in FY 1999 (FCS, 2000, Minutes of the Board of Directors).

Daily Life Support Service

Home Help and Care Service. The service includes bathing and toileting in addition to ordinary home help services for cooking, cleaning, shopping, and so forth.

The operators of the service are workers' collectives called "Helpers." They operate in a small residential area, or across a ward of a city or town. The main groups and strata receiving help and services from the associations are: the elderly, people with health problems, and low-income families. These recipients are informed about the activities of the Helper mainly through personal contact and via the public relations of the association. On occasions, the assistance of the local government and other non-profit organization is useful (Oka, 2000b, p. 32).

A local coordinator of the Helpers visits the people on request and recommends joining the FCS. There is almost no test or assessment by which it is decided who should be helped. Those who agree to accept the rules of FCS and pay a small membership fee can join the FCS (Oka, 2000b, p. 33; interview with Mr. Yokota, 2001).

All associations provide service against payment–the so-called "Community Price." Theoretically, FCS explains it as a price for the provisional settlement between caregiving members and care-receiving members. In the longer perspective, FCS expects today's caregivers to receive care services from other members. Practically, it means that the labor cost is lower than the market price, and other costs are approximately the same as the actual expenses. The Community Price is currently 840 yen ($7) per hour for daytime of weekdays, and 1,260 yen ($10.5) per hour for nighttime and holidays. This is considerably cheaper than the ordinary market price (Oka, 2000b, p. 34; interview with Mr. Hamada, 2001).

The home help and care service started in 1987 with one Helper and 26 members. Because the low-price policy did not include the cost of service-coordinators, it suffered from deficit. Since 1993, when the FCS board decided to support the Helpers with surplus from the goods delivery service, the business has been developing rapidly. Between FY 1994 and 2000, the Helpers increased from four bodies with a membership of 213 to nine bodies with a membership of 570. Their total annual sales increased 12.5 times from 9 million yen ($75,000) to 112 million yen ($937,000). Helpers Collectives served 728 member-customers of FCS with a total of 83,200 service hours as of FY 2000. On average, each member of Helpers worked approximately 146 hours and earned 126,000 yen ($1,050) per year. It can be estimated that a caregiving member served a care-receiving member once a week for 2-3 hours (see Tables 2 and 3).

Meals-On-Wheels Service. The service aims at responding to the needs of the elderly for whom cooking is difficult or troublesome. The needs were identified through the activities of Caretakers and Helpers.

TABLE 3. Performance of Workers' Collectives for Life Support Services (FY 2000)

	Home help and care service	Meals-on-wheels service	Transportation service	Total
1) No. of W.Co.	9	4	1	14
2) Caregivers	570	82	12	664
3) Care-receivers	728	474	64	1,266
4) Service hours	83,200	79,000	565	162,765
5) Invested-capital	¥16,400 $136,700	¥7,750 $64,600	¥830 $6,917	¥24,980 $208,200
6) Sales/service-charges	¥112,400 $936,700	¥81,000 $675,000	¥1,550 $12,900	¥194,950 $1,624,600
7) Pay to caregivers	¥72,000 $600,000	¥32,920 $274,300	¥1,120 $9,300	¥106,040 $883,700

Note:
* ¥: Japanese 1,000 Yen. $: U.S. Dollar. The exchange rate: $1 = 120 Yen.
1) No. of W.Co.: Number of workers' collective associations.
2) Caregivers: The members of workers' collectives engaged in caregiving services.
3) Care-receivers: Member-customers or service users of FCS.
Source: Calculated from the Minutes of FCS Board of Directors, 2001.

The workers' collectives engaging in the meals-on-wheels service are very sensitive to the use of additive-free ingredients and balanced nutrition. Recently, they started a special service for diabetics, for persons with liver disorders, and for other special needs. They cook and deliver meals in the evenings, Monday through Saturday. Those who deliver the meals carefully monitor the member-customers and make contact with relevant persons/institutions if necessary (Oka, 2000b, p. 39).

The price of a meal is 900 yen ($7.5). According to the cost accounting of FCS, the cost of a meal is 1,320 yen ($11). This includes 420 yen ($3.5) for the personnel expenses, 350 yen ($2.9) for the material cost and 550 yen ($4.6) for non-personnel expenses. FCS has requested public support but has been unsuccessful to date (FCS, 2001, Minutes of the Board of Directors).

The service started in 1994 at one workers' collective with 15 members. The annual sales were only 1.2 million yen ($10,000). As of FY 2000, there were four workers' collectives with a membership of 82 that included 14 qualified persons such as nutritionists and hygiene specialists. They served 474 member-customers with a total of 93,600 meals.

The annual sales were 81 million yen ($675,000), and the total working hours were 79,000. On average, a member of the workers' collective worked 963 hours and received 400,000 yen ($3,300) a year. It can be estimated that a member-customer received the service three to four times a week (see Tables 2 and 3).

Transportation Service. The service aims at responding to the needs of elderly persons who want to enjoy the outdoor life, including leisure activities, shopping, and so forth. The service started in FY 2000 with a workers' collective with 12 members. They bought a vehicle from donations at a welfare festival hosted by FCS.

Customers pay 1,500 yen ($12.5) for the annual membership fee. The basic service charge for the first hour is 1,500 yen ($12.5), and then 500 yen ($4.2) is added for every 30 minutes. In the evenings and holidays, an extra charge of 250 yen ($2.1) is added for every 30 minutes. The gas charge is 40 yen ($0.3) per one kilometer. In the case of two hours of service during the daytime of a weekday, the total charge would be approximately 3,000 yen ($25), less than half of the cost of hiring a taxi (interview with Mr. Hamada, 2001).

In FY 2000, 64 member-customers used the service for 565 hours. On average, a member-customer used the service three to four times a year. The sales were 1.6 million yen ($12,900) as shown in Table 3. The net pay for the drivers was 800 yen ($6.7) per hour. On average, a member of the workers' collective worked 47 hours and earned 38,000 yen ($317) in the year. In FY 2001, a further workers' collective was inaugurated. The total membership of the two associations increased to 30. This included one care-manager and 15 qualified home-helpers (FCS, 2001, Minutes of the Board of Directors).

Housing and Facility Services

The third pillar of FCS is the construction of small complexes of buildings that combine adequate homes and care facilities for the elderly in their community. It aims to provide comfortable homes with care services as well as community spaces in which the elderly can enjoy their lives with rich human contact (FCS, 2000, pp. 50-51).

To implement the idea, FCS started research in 1990 and presented a tentative plan in 1995. A member of FCS, Mrs. Ishida, positively responded to the project. She wanted FCS to utilize her property to build an ideal facility. She expressed her desire in a phrase: "Trust and live together" (FCS, 2000, pp. 48-49).

Responding to the offer, FCS immediately established a project team. In the spring of 1998, final agreement was reached between FCS and Mrs. Ishida. The first and second floors of the three-story building would be used for the day service while the third floor would be Mrs. Ishida's private home. Mrs. Ishida would retain the ownership of the whole building and the land site, and FCS would rent the first and second floors at 300,000 yen ($2,500) per month. Mrs. Ishida promised to donate the whole property to FCS on her death. The total construction cost of the building was approximately 110 million yen ($917,000) of which Mrs. Ishida agreed to pay 80 million yen ($667,000). FCS agreed to spend 30 million yen ($250,000) on the cost of the interior decoration of the day service floors (FCS, 2000, pp. 50-51; interview with Ms. Iwaki, 2000).

Prior to construction, FCS organized a workers' collective to provide the day service in the facility. The 18 members were middle-aged housewives wanting to engage in meaningful work in their community. They developed their caregiving skills through training as well as their own concepts of desirable care. They insisted that the most important issue was to guarantee each client time to relax in the facility with freedom of choice. They also promised that all information about the facility should be disclosed for further development of a social and community-based health service (FCS, 2000, pp. 46-47).

The facility's opening in May 1999 attracted considerable public attention as the first experiment utilizing private property for the semi-public day service. The service was available from 10 a.m. to 3 p.m., Monday through Friday. The service included recreation activities, rehabilitation, bathing, lunch service, transportation service to and from the facility, and a comprehensive consulting service for clients and their family members. The clients were mostly 80-90 years of age, and they joined FCS for a small membership fee. It was reported that the homely atmosphere in the facility was so effective for a client with senile dementia that his mental condition improved (FCS, 2000; interview with Ms. Iwaki, 2000).

During the start-up phase of the facility between May 1999 and March 2000, the local government of Kamakura City played an important role. It contracted out the day service with 25.5 million yen ($212,500), which amounted to 95% of the total income. In addition, the local government granted 3.5 million yen ($29,167) for two vehicles.

FCS currently plans to build a similar facility in Yokohama City in the near future (FCS, 2001, Minutes of the Board of Directors).

SOCIAL SERVICE REFORM AND FCS

In April 2000, a new long-term care insurance system called Public Personal Care Insurance was inaugurated. Insured persons aged 40 or over pay a premium, and the national and local governments contribute the same amount. The insurers and administrators of the insurance system are the local governments. The reform symbolized the conversion of the Japanese social service system from a paternalistic one to a market-oriented system.

In the preparatory stage of the new system, the leaders of FCS were seriously concerned about sustainability of their movement, because large profit-making enterprises were expected to participate in the new attractive market and to expel small-scale non-profit business. However, since the beneficiaries of the insurance system would be only 10% to 15% of the population aged 65 and over due to strict assessment of care needs, they understood that their service might still be necessary for the non-beneficiaries. They also decided to participate in the insurance system as a service provider to ensure the system is continuously based on people's needs that could be discovered through daily activities at workers' collectives (interview with Mr. K. Yokota, 2001).

The strategy of FCS to cope with the new insurance system consisted of three elements. The first concerned how to establish a healthy basis for a non-profit business. It was necessary to reconsider the low-price policy that could afford neither the cost of service coordinators nor the fund for further development of workers' collectives. The outcome of fierce debates was that FCS decided to raise the charge of the home help and care service gradually from 840 yen ($7) to 1,140 yen ($9.5) per hour by FY 2002. At the same time, FCS made an appeal to local governments to enact a bylaw aimed at supporting workers' collectives with stable subsidies and grants. However, this has not been realized yet. The second element was how to establish an organizational structure that could meet the requirements of the new insurance system. A legal-person status was required for officially authorized service providers, but this was very difficult for small workers' collectives to do. To cope with this situation, FCS established new legal-persons in five areas of the Kanagawa Prefecture in collaboration with the SCSK group. These five organizations, qualified as official service providers, have contracted out actual care services to Helpers workers' collectives. The third point was how to improve the quality of care services. This was necessary for enhancing competitiveness as well as meeting legal requirements concerning the quality of the caregiving work force. Aiming to meet the challenge, FCS established a training system that enabled the members of workers' collectives to obtain officially authorized qualifications as home helpers and in care services (SCSK, 2000, pp. 133-161, 178-193).

What were the effects of the new insurance system for FCS? In FY 1999-2000, the number of Helpers collectives remained at nine, and their total membership increased from 546 to 570. However, business performance showed a remarkable improvement (see Tables 2 and 3).

The total service hours of home help and care service increased 21% from 68,660 to 83,200, which was divided equally between the beneficiaries of the new insurance system and non-beneficiaries. Total sales increased 157% from 44 million yen ($367,000) to 112 million yen ($933,000), of which 70% was earned from services for beneficiaries of the new insurance system (FCS, 2001, Minutes of the Board of Directors).

From FY 1999-2000, the pay to actual caregiving members remained at 700-800 yen ($5.8-6.7) per hour. On average, the earnings of each worker increased from 92,000 yen ($770) to 126,000 yen ($1,050) (FCS, 2001, Minutes of the Board of Directors; interview with Mr. Hamada, 2001).

The new insurance system paid the following per hour: 1,600 yen ($13.3) for the standard home help service, 4,300 yen ($35.8) for body-contact care services, and 2,900 yen ($24.2) for a medium service between the two. The difference between the above-mentioned public price and the service cost of FCS was pooled and utilized as funds for further development of FCS and workers' collectives. The new insurance system gave FCS an important opportunity to improve the business performance of workers' collectives engaging in home help and care services.

The new insurance system also stimulated FCS to improve the quality of the care service. As of FY 2000, the members of Helpers included nine care managers, 13 nurses, 242 officially qualified home helpers, and other specialists such as social workers. The total number of qualified persons was 271 or 48% of the total membership (FCS, 2001, Minutes of the Board of Directors). According to a survey, the percentage was less than 10% as of FY 1998 (Oka, M., 2000b, p. 38). It suggests the progress of Helpers from a non-professional group towards a mix of professionals and non-professionals.

On the other hand, the new insurance system caused some difficulties for FCS. Some experienced caregiving members chose to start their own home help businesses or to engage in jobs in private companies with better pay than that of workers' collectives. While the number of members who have left is few to date, this may present a major challenge to FCS and the workers' collectives in the future (interview with Ms. Iwaki, 2000).

CONCLUDING REMARKS

This section summarizes the contributions of FCS toward a welfare community.

The Quantitative Contribution

FCS has successively organized homemakers into workers' collectives and developed various services over the past 10 years. The list of available services shows that a comprehensive range of services is provided. The home delivery service of goods has been very convenient for frail member-customers to fulfill their fundamental needs for healthy and successful aging. In FY 2000, FCS organized 670 homemakers for this service in nine workers' collectives called Caretakers and delivered goods worth 2.7 billion yen ($22.6 million). Moreover, this service included a caretaking service. The delivery members have carefully watched the situation of approximately 13,000 member-customers and have provided useful information as well as stopgap services. The value of this caretaking service cannot be estimated in monetary terms. In combination with the delivery service, FCS has identified the needs of the elderly and enriched the service menu through the daily activities of workers' collectives and their networks. As a result, the workers' collectives engaged in the life support services provided a total of 163,000 hours of service worth 195 million yen ($1.6 million) in FY 2000. They successfully organized 664 homemakers to work in providing home help and other related services, and provided these services to 1,266 members of FCS at a very small charge. While the number of care-receiving members looks small compared to the member-customers of delivery service, it is increasing rapidly. Thus, the quantitative contribution of the services has been considerable (see Tables 1, 2, and 3).

The Qualitative Contribution

The workers' collectives have provided flexible and complex services for supporting the daily lives of the elderly based on the experience and wisdom of homemakers. According to a senior civil servant of a local government, their human-touch service is in sharp contrast to bureaucratic public services and profitmaking private services (Gáthy & Széman, 2000, pp. 27-28).

A Model for an Alternative Social Service System

FCS's creative activities, based on the spirit of mutual help and social solidarity, clearly indicate a positive role for the non-profit sector. This inexpensive and high-quality service has successfully competed against profitmaking organizations in the care-service market and has promoted improvements of public services. The donated building to offer shelter to frail members has functioned as a combination of housing/community day center. It is the first such experiment in Japan and echoes the bed and care homes in the United States. (See "Housing and Facility Services" in this article.)

FCS has also been successful in socializing unpaid work and creating valuable job opportunities for women. Their annual earnings can be estimated between 100,000 and 400,000 yen ($830-3,300). This was far lower than the upper limit of the tax-free income of 1.03 million yen ($8,600) for homemakers of the salaried class. Therefore, the earnings are only a supplementary income for their families. Nonetheless, FCS has made a considerable contribution to the local economy as well as to women in terms of opening the gate to take part in useful work in the community. The total invested capital by members, more than 500 million yen ($4.2 million), also shows their great contribution to the accumulation of social capital. FCS has utilized it as a fund for enlarging its activities and improving services. The civil initiative presented by FCS and the workers' collectives suggests a possibility of a community-based social service system that may guarantee quality services without raising tax and premiums for social insurance.

The public long-term care insurance system, started in FY 2000, has caused both positive and negative effects to FCS, as mentioned earlier. In the near future, the market-oriented insurance system will force FCS to compete against profitmaking service-providers. To cope with this challenge, FCS plans to develop a comprehensive consulting service for both beneficiaries and non-beneficiaries of the new insurance system. FCS also plans to organize a volunteer network of senior citizens including its members as well as non-members who cannot join the workers' collectives for various reasons, but want to make a contribution to the community. FCS expects that these new measures will be effective for obtaining rich information on actual needs and developing an effective mutual support system among community members (FCS, Minutes of Board of Directors, 2001).

Replication of FCS Elsewhere in Japan and in Other Societies

In Japan, some consumer cooperatives recently started home delivery service of goods. However, the majority outsourced the provision of the service to private companies due to difficulties in organizing workers' collectives. Because of personnel resources grown up in the joint purchase activities of the SCSK group over the past 30 years, FCS has been able to achieve this. It would not be easy to replicate FCS in the short-term.

Regarding the home help service, there were 165 workers' collectives in Japan as of FY 1999 (SCSK, 2000, pp. 198-213). This shows the potential for replication of FCS. However, many problems must be solved to stimulate further development of the workers' collective movement (SCSK, 2000, pp. 121-123; Kanagawa Workers' Collective Rengo Kai, 2000, pp. 103-108).

First, many workers' collectives currently cannot obtain legal-person's status due to strict conditions defined by the NPO (non-profit organization) Act of 1998. As a result, they can neither hold possession of their own collective properties nor make contracts directly with local governments and other relevant bodies. Moreover, tax concessions are not available to them. Therefore, a reform of the NPO Act and related laws is crucial.

Second, most of the workers' collectives are financially poor. They often suffer from a shortage of funds to maintain and develop their activities. Therefore, it is necessary for local governments to enact bylaws that guarantee stable public support to workers' collectives.

Third, currently, the members of workers' collectives are not entitled to public insurance for on-the-job accidents and other public compensation systems. It is necessary to establish relevant social security measures for such groups of workers.

Workers' collectives should also implement specific new policies. For example, it might be crucial to establish an effective training system aimed at enhancing members' caregiving skills. It is also necessary to strengthen the solidarity of the workers' collective movement in order to promote its development further.

FCS has successfully resolved some of these issues in collaboration with the SCSK Movement Group as a whole. If the cooperative movement could successfully meet this agenda, workers' collectives might play a further important role in the social services of 21st century Japan.

With regard to the international perspective, FCS appears to share the common values with the "Time Dollars" approach, especially in terms of "Reciprocity" and "Redefining Work" (Cahn, 2000). Further, the idea of FCS combining middle-aged and older members in one organization echoes the work by Edgar Cahn. While FCS does not use a Time Yen, the Community Price approach of FCS is essentially the same idea as the "Time Dollars" approach in terms of providing a useful measure for promoting a reciprocal support system among neighborhood community members (Time Dollar Institute, 2001). It suggests a potential for international solidarity and cooperation among non-profit organizations that share common values for rebuilding a good community, based on active participation of citizens.

AUTHOR NOTES

Masato Oka is Professor and Director at the Economic Research Institute, Yokohama City University, Yokohama, Japan. He is co-author of *Regulating Employment and Welfare: Company and National Policies of Labor Force Participation at the End of Worklife in Industrial Countries* and *Advancing Aging Policy as the 21st Century Begins*. He was Guest Editor of a 1996 issue of the *Journal of Aging & Social Policy* (Vol. 8, Nos. 2/3) on public policy and the old-age revolution in Japan.

Professor Oka can be contacted at Yokohama City University, Economic Research Institute, 22-2 Seto, Kanazawa-ku, Yokohama, Japan, 236-0027 (E-mail: okamasat@yokohama-cu.ac.jp).

REFERENCES

Cahn, E. (2000). *No more throw-away people: The co-production imperative.* Washington, DC: Essential Book.

FCS (2000). *Workers' collective ga tukuru tiiki fukusi: Fukushi Club Seikyo no 10 nen* (Community welfare created by workers' collectives: Ten years history of FCS). Yokohama: Author. (In Japanese).

FCS (1999-2001). Minutes of the Board of Directors and attached reports. Unpublished manuscripts. (In Japanese).

Gáthy, V., & Széman, Z. (Eds.) (2000). *Challenges in the ageing societies of Japan and Hungary: The role of nonprofit organizations.* Budapest and Yokohama: Institute of Sociology, Hungarian Academy of Sciences, and Economic Research Institute, Yokohama City University.

Kanagawa Workers' Collective Rengo Kai (Workers' Collective Kanagawa Union) (Ed.) (2000). *Josei to Shimin ga hiraku atarashii jidai: Kanagawa Workers' Collective Rengo Kai no 10 nen no ayumi* (A new age created by women and citizens:

Ten years history of the Workers' Collective Kanagawa Union). Yokohama: Author. (In Japanese).

Oka, M. (2000a). A special consumer cooperative association nursing home. *Journal of Aging & Social Policy*, *11*(2/3), 99-106.

Oka, M. (2000b). A survey on Japan's workers' collective associations serving the elderly. In V. Gáthy and Z. Széman (Eds.), *Op. Cit.* (pp. 29-41).

SCSK (Ed.) (1991). *Ikiiki alternative: Seikatsu Club Kanagawa 20 nen no ayumi* (Twenty years history of SCSK). Yokohama: Author. (In Japanese).

SCSK Movement Group (Ed.) (2000). *Sanka gata fukushi shakai wo hiraku* (Creating a participatory welfare community). Tokyo: Fuhdosha. (In Japanese).

Time Dollar Institute (2001). 'What are Time Dollars and how do they work?' in Timedollar Website: (*http://www.timedollar.org/101/x1Question one.htm*).

Yokota, K. (1991). *I among others*. Tokyo: Seikatsu Club. (In English).

INTERVIEWS

Mr. Hamada, Koji (managing director of FCS). October 2001.
Ms. Iwaki, Kayoko (head of Day Ishida). November 2000.
Ms. Ogawa, Yasuko (head of Rapport Fujisawa). September 2001.
Ms. Tagawa, Motoko (head of FCS). October 2001.
Mr. Yokota, Katsumi (former head of FCS, the leader of SCSK group). September 2001.

ACKNOWLEDGEMENTS

The above-named interviewees and other members of FCS and SCSK group gave full support to the research. The Yokohama City University and the Univers Foundation granted generous financial support. The author would like to express sincere thanks for these supports.

Kaiser Permanente's Manifesto 2005 Demonstration: The Promises and Limits of Devolution

Walter Leutz, PhD
Brandeis University

Merwyn Greenlick, PhD
Oregon Health & Sciences University

Lucy Nonnenkamp, MA
Richard della Penna, MD
Kaiser Permanente

SUMMARY. In 1996, the eight-million member Kaiser Permanente HMO adopted a vision statement that said by 2005 it would expand its services to include home- and community-based services for its members with disabilities. It funded a 3-year, 32-site demonstration that showed that it was feasible to link HMO services with existing home- and community-based (HCB) services and that members appreciated the improved coordination and access. This private-sector project showed that devolution can produce innovative and feasible models of care, but it also showed that without federal financial and regulatory support, such models are unlikely to take hold if they are focused on "unprofitable"

[Haworth co-indexing entry note]: "Kaiser Permanente's Manifesto 2005 Demonstration: The Promises and Limits of Devolution." Leutz, Walter et al. Co-published simultaneously in *Journal of Aging & Social Policy* (The Haworth Press, Inc.) Vol. 14, No. 3/4, 2002, pp. 233-244; and: *Devolution and Aging Policy* (ed: Francis G. Caro, and Robert Morris) The Haworth Press, Inc., 2002, pp. 233-244. Single or multiple copies of this article are available for a fee from The Haworth Document Delivery Service [1-800-HAWORTH, 9:00 a.m. - 5:00 p.m. (EST). E-mail address: getinfo@haworthpressinc.com].

10.1300/J031v14n03_13

populations, for example, those who are chronically ill, poor, and/or disabled. *[Article copies available for a fee from The Haworth Document Delivery Service: 1-800-HAWORTH. E-mail address: <getinfo@haworthpressinc.com> Website: <http://www.HaworthPress.com> © 2002 by The Haworth Press, Inc. All rights reserved.]*

KEYWORDS. Managed care, home care, care management, integration

DESCRIPTION OF A DEVOLVED DEMONSTRATION

In September 1997, the Kaiser Permanente health care system (KP) launched a demonstration of home- and community-based support services (community care) for members with disabilities. The demonstration was inspired by KP's experience with the Social HMO (Greenlick et al., 1988; Leutz et al., 1994) and Model of Care (Marshall et al., 1999) demonstrations, as well as other initiatives of its national aging network. Funded by $2 million in KP funds, the purpose of the three-year demonstration was to develop and test models for implementing Manifesto 2005, a vision statement adopted by KP leadership in 1996:

> By the year 2005, KP will have expanded its scope of services to include a broad range of home- and community-based services that will be easily accessible to persons with functional disabilities. This will be a multidisciplinary system with providers and consumers of care working in collaboration to maximize the independent function of persons with disabilities of any age.

The Manifesto 2005 initiative was unusual–if not unique–in two ways. First, KP was showing interest in the community services aspects of chronic illness and disabilities, not just the medical care aspects. Many models for providing better medical care have been demonstrated (Kramer et al., 1992), but significant improvements in standard practice are needed to change system performance (Splaine et al., 1998), including moving to redress the balance of care toward a public health model (Kutza, 1997). The second unusual aspect was KP's spending $2 million of its own funds to develop and test a new model outside of its traditional service boundaries. The potential for acute care savings was an interest, but not the primary one. More important were meeting staff desires to serve members' needs better.

The 32 sites participating in the demonstration were chosen from nearly 200 applications. They represented a broad range of community care services to be connected to the KP system of care. At almost all sites, the approach to adding community care services was not to add these services as benefits but to "link" and "coordinate" medical care with existing community care (Leutz, 1999). The planning group saw this as a broader and more practical alternative to collaborating than the "integration" models being tested in other national initiatives, which generally required enrolling new populations, assuming risk for an expanded range of services, and acquiring special waivers from Medicare and/or Medicaid (Wiener & Skaggs, 1995). In contrast, linkage and coordination take medical and community care systems as they are and try to make them work better together. They do not require waivers, contracts, multidisciplinary teams, or financing new benefits. But they do require medical and community systems to do something that they seldom do now, that is, work together on a personal, real-time basis around helping individuals served in both systems. Most of the onus for action rests with the medical system, but there are also things community care can do.

Linkage is the simpler way to connect medical and community care, and linkage may be enough for individuals with simple or stable community care needs, or who are able to self-manage, or who have strong family supports. To initiate linkage, medical care needs to understand who pays for what and who is eligible for what in community care, and to have staff that can make appropriate referrals to community care agencies and follow up on those referrals. Linkage also includes identifying patients who may need community care through publicity, screening, and internal referral systems in medical care. This includes getting clinicians to talk about disability and community care with their patients. Implied in this is the need to create understanding among clinicians of the value of community services to their patients.

Coordination builds on linkage by adding, first, a care management function in the medical system, and second, more explicit understandings with community care agencies. Ideally, there is an analogous care management function to coordinate community care services. Coordination may be needed for individuals who use multiple community care services, whose medical conditions are unstable or complex, and whose informal support systems need help. A coordinated system more actively informs medical providers about community care needs and services, facilitates transitions across settings, and receives and provides input for physicians and other providers. A coordinated system also negotiates guidelines and agreements between medical and community care agencies for making and accepting referrals, for who will pay for what to maximize efficiency and coverage, and for what information will be shared about clients and care plans. Coordination is generally what first-round Social HMOs do, but they also finance new community care services, which is a bonus but not a requirement for coordination. Coordination also provides a structure through which both parties can reliably collaborate in care, planning, expansion, etc.

Since some of the 32 KP demonstration sites were combined into multi-site projects, in the end there were 15 distinct projects, all of which furthered community care connections. Projects tested linkages to adaptive technology for members of all ages, community care services for a newly enrolled SSI Medicaid population, early intervention for infants and young children, and adult day services, personal care, and transportation for elders. One multi-site linkage project developed volunteer programs for social support, and another developed caregiver-training classes. Members were linked to both.

There were also coordination projects. One multi-site project developed a protocol for post-diagnosis dementia care that coordinated services with local Alzheimer's Association chapters. Another developed and tested a protocol to coordinate care for members in adult foster homes.

Not all were linkage and coordination. Two sites extended KP benefits to home care aides for members who do not qualify for skilled home health care. There were also information-gathering projects. One conducted group and individual interviews with caregivers and members with disabilities to understand their experiences accessing health and community care services. Another analyzed administrative and clinical data systems to try to identify members with disabilities.

The Manifesto 2005 initiative explored a new idea: connecting a managed medical system to community care across a range of populations and services. The new territory–along with the limited funding available to any single project–made the research design more akin to a series of reconnaissance missions than a coordinated set of scientific experiments. The missions were essentially feasibility studies focusing on the structure, process, and outputs of projects. This type of approach provides information that is both usable for and believable to the managers of medical care programs. They see fair approximations of the costs, staffing, persons served, and impacts in projects that are actually operating in their service settings.

Although project applicants were not required to hypothesize or test impacts on patient health status or on health services utilization or costs, each project had its own particular set of research questions. Answering these contributed to answering the overall question being addressed in the demonstration: What approaches can KP use to understand better the needs and wants of its members with disabilities and to connect them more effectively to community care supports? Related questions included:

- How many KP members had particular disabilities, what were their needs, and how could these members be identified?
- What were the ranges of community care services these members used?
- How could KP staff coordinate with and support community care providers, including informal caregivers?
- What were the costs, benefits, and barriers to extending KP activities into community care services?
- How could successful projects be sustained and replicated?

Although the demonstration for the most part did not use controlled research designs, it did gather data on common elements, including quarterly reports on operational progress and problems, a baseline Health Status Form (HSF) from participants based on the form KP uses in its Social HMO and Medicare+Choice programs (Brody et al., 1997), and aggregate utilization data on the services provided. Additionally, most of the group sites assessed at least some aspects of their impacts on participants, including overall satisfaction with project services and pre-post differences in areas such as learning through project services and changes in community care service use. A few of the larger sites had sufficient sample sizes to explore questions about differential impacts by participant characteristics or by individual site.

The demonstration evaluation identified a basic linkage model followed by almost every site. It included four internal structures and processes to coordinate and link with community care:

- A single point of contact within KP for providers, community agencies, and members to call to give and obtain information. A nurse or social worker usually staffed this.
- Training for KP providers in how to identify and refer potential community care users to the point of contact.
- Outreach to members and families to let them know why and how to get help.

- Information systems to help KP providers track the basic facts about community care referrals, caregivers, and functional issues.

Details of the sites' experiences and a proposal for a mature linkage and coordination system are found in a forthcoming book on the demonstration (Leutz et al., 2002).

DEVOLUTION AND THE MANIFESTO 2005 DEMONSTRATION

The concept of "devolution" is for the federal government to give more responsibility for shaping and paying for health and social welfare services to states, localities, and the private sector. Manifesto 2005 demonstration was in many ways an archetype for devolution–a national initiative by a private organization to address a pressing health and human services issue in innovative ways. There are a number of ways in which the KP experience supports devolution as a development and implementation model. But the demonstration also shows the limitations of devolution–at least in improving services for people with disabilities. The following section reflects on ways that devolution seemed to work well, while the second part argues that, ultimately, devolution as a policy in this service area is likely to fail without getting some support "from above."

How Devolution Worked Well

The private sector stepped forward. KP showed that the private (non-profit) sector is capable of taking initiative to do something special for elders and others with disabilities. They acted on their perceptions of their members' needs and their own prior experiences with approaches for addressing needs to develop a new vision and model of care. Because this was a need they felt, the project had credibility in the system, and staff that most felt the need stepped forward to participate with enthusiasm and relevant experience.

The model fit the organization. The initiative that was developed fit the KP system. The managers and clinicians in KP's aging network knew how to move the national system, and the individual site leaders had similar local knowledge. Because they designed the project, it worked for them. The demonstration leadership got institutional and financial support from health plan and medical group leadership. Then, they used their inter-regional committees and networks to start, publicize, and implement the project.

The model allowed local variation. Within the system-wide framework, the project allowed for local variation. This was important, both within KP and to accommodate different community care systems. In the multi-site projects, different KP units took the lead at different sites, in part because regions were organized differently and in part because the individuals most interested came from different departments. Similarly, the community agencies that participated differed. For example, in the multi-site volunteer project, three of the sites had faith-based partners, one partnered with a service agency, and three sites used KP volunteers.

Community care agencies participated. Consistent with KP's interest in improving the care system, community care providers and public interest organizations (e.g., Alzheimer's Association) were ready and able partners. Although there were clear service gaps (see limits of devolution below), they had important services to offer individuals with disabilities and families. Improved information about community care services and facilitated access to them were highly valued by members. These capabilities were worked out locally through meetings, in-service training, and development of personal relationships. In some projects, local participation was also facilitated by support from national organizations.

One devolved element that was missing was participation by public agencies. Aside from the one site focused on enrolling SSI beneficiaries and another that received encouragement from a state unit on aging, site leaders neither asked for nor received any particular help from public sector managers or policymakers. This is one element that we recommend folding into expanded efforts, since states and localities certainly have an interest in strengthening linkage and coordination.

The costs were modest. The costs of setting up and operating linkage and coordination systems were relatively modest. The major staff cost was the single point of contact in the medical system, and an analogous staff person would exist in an organized community care system. Other costs were information system enhancements to track the status of service users and outreach/advertising. With the exception of two home care benefit expansions within KP, projects did not add funding for community care services. It seemed that most people were able to find the community care support they needed, and the linkage systems helped them connect.

There were paybacks in goodwill. Members and families noticed and appreciated KP's efforts, and so did community agency staff–and of course KP staff gained an appreciation of community care partners.

Thus, the projects showed the potential of generating the kind of local political and customer support that are essential for a devolved care system.

The model worked for all groups. The need for better linkage cut across age and disability groups, and the models for connecting were very similar, even though the specific community agencies and the internal KP departments differed. The issues and approaches were very much "devolved" ones: understanding how particular programs worked and could be accessed, establishing personal and referral relationships, reaching out to potential users, educating providers, etc.

The model could be adapted for other systems. The approaches that KP tested for linking medical care and community care are relevant to other managed care settings and also could be adopted for fee-for-service settings. The problems of poor connections and communications between medical care and community care systems are virtually universal. Although national directives for better connections would help, in the end, the connections need to be made locally–agency by agency, practice by practice–taking into account the strengths, weaknesses, and peculiarities of local systems. As an organized medical care system, KP was able relatively easily to marshal participation from key players (e.g., primary care physicians, associated specialists, discharge planning, home health). Less integrated health plans would need to work harder, and perhaps community-wide approaches would be the logical outcome. This would require public sector leadership and support, as discussed below. Finally, although this was not tested in the demonstration, it is reasonable to think that the model would work for coordinating other services used by people of all ages with serious chronic illness–with or without functional disability.

How Devolution Is Likely to Fail

Although there was much in the KP demonstration to support devolution, the experience also poses serious questions about pure devolution as a strategy for widespread and lasting change. The questions revolve mostly around money: who would invest in startup and ongoing costs? Will there be returns on investment and who will reap those returns? Will these investments and benefits serve public or private purposes? There is also the nagging question of inadequate community care infrastructure and service funding. Of course, how these questions are answered differs by whether devolution is seen as a purely private initiative or whether local or state governments participate. We will look at the private side first.

How much can you count on private initiative? The $2 million KP invested in the Manifesto 2005 demonstration actually started off as $3 million, but one year into the demonstration, that figure was cut by a third due to system-wide losses and budget cuts. That is still a good deal of money, and $2 million (plus a lot of local KP in-kind contributions) was enough to support a meaningful demonstration. Nevertheless, the fact of the cut shows the precariousness of reliance on private investment in R&D.

In a market-based health care system, the reason an organization would make R&D investments is in anticipation that eventually they will reduce costs, increase net revenues, or improve the product enough to increase market share and net revenues. We were not able to even argue (let alone prove) that linking with community care would save money directly for KP or make money otherwise because it tapped a lucrative market. There is not much other demonstration evidence that community care can substitute for medical care services, and arguing that this would take place would not have been a strong inducement for community providers to participate. Several were already reported to be suspicious that KP was trying to get them to do its work.

Moreover, people with disabilities are among the poorest, sickest, and most difficult members for health care systems to serve. Thus, this was hardly a market with enhanced revenue potential, unless KP had somehow targeted only to members who could pay for the extra attention, which would have been inimical to the plan's mission. On top of this, the business and marketing managers could point to data that show it is bad business to make your plan more attractive to people with disabilities. Therefore, even improving access and health outcomes for these high-cost groups (which are plausible results) would not be a good market reason to invest in linkage. Most of the projects ended after the demonstration, because local budgets did not pick up the costs for maintaining linkage.

Another way to develop a successful private initiative for sick and low-income people is for these groups' public insurers (Medicare and Medicaid) to pay for the extra system capabilities. This has been the approach of several decades of Medicare and Medicaid demonstrations, including most recently the state dual eligible initiatives, which offer a way for managed care organizations to become responsible for medical care, community care, and even long-term institutional care for beneficiaries with chronic illnesses and disabilities. One problem with this from a devolution perspective is that reliance on national entitlement programs to make local and private initiatives work stretches the meaning of "devolution." Another problem is that so far the "devolved" integration initiatives have been very complex to develop and operate. Yet another is that they include only people who are eligible for these entitlements, while the KP demonstration model can be available to all members with disabilities, regardless of income, funding, or level or type of disability.

Can the local public sector pick up devolution? The argument for a state or local public investment in linkage/coordination is stronger than the case for private interest. The public model is based on old-fashioned public health, creating an infrastructure that helps all people with disabilities and their families, which would in turn create a wide net of public interest in the system. This is a compelling vision, but there are some major bridges to build before we get there.

First, where should the money come from? Is it new expenditures (hard to find) or a redistribution of current ones (hard to sell)? Even if new money is found, under-funded community care service systems can make strong cases that services themselves should be funded first or as well. These types of dilemmas make heads turn to richer federal sources, which also bring red tape to patch up local turf battles.

Second, the KP linkage projects connected many people in the KP demonstration to services, but the projects also exposed community care shortcomings. Even in the relatively "good" communities and states where most demonstration sites operated (CA, CO, HI, OR), the typical weaknesses of community care in the United States hampered efforts: The services were too expensive for some members; others were blocked by waiting lists; many agencies lacked the staff and systems to coordinate and cooperate; and local service systems were usually fragmented. A serious effort to link medical care and community care would likely fail if access to basic community care services were a continuing obstacle.

How about a local public/private partnership? The KP aging network leadership is considering a second-phase demonstration model that asks local KP service areas (serving about 500,000 members or less) to get together with community care providers and local and state government to propose how they would demonstrate a mature linkage and coordination system available to all individuals with disabilities. Support for the project would ideally include foundation funds for start-up and evaluation, new local public funds to fill gaps in community care systems, and a modest increment to the HMO capitation (e.g., a dime a member a month) to support KP efforts. Of course, this could be expanded to include other HMOs/communities or even medical care and community care systems that are not based on HMOs.

We are hopeful that we can find funds for this second-generation test of a "mature" linkage and coordination model and that a KP service area and its community will demonstrate real improvements in access, quality, satisfaction, etc. Creating this kind of system is definitely a local project, and if it succeeded it would seem to make the case for devolution. But would it? Where would the project go from there without federal money and supportive policy? Perhaps some additional enlightened or wealthy states or localities within states would also act, which would be good for people who live there, but this would also increase the already existing inequalities in services for people with disabilities. Without a federal commitment to support models of local control and initiative that work, devolution alone is unlikely to serve public health interests of all people with disabilities, including elders.

AUTHOR NOTES

Walter Leutz is Associate Professor at Brandeis University's Heller School, where he teaches courses in long-term care. He is Director of the Social HMO Consortium, a university-provider cooperative that has developed, expanded, and researched a managed care model for integrating acute and long-term care services for Medicare beneficiaries. He was also Research Director of the system-wide Kaiser Permanente demonstration of how to add community long-term care services to the Kaiser Permanente clinical continuum. Dr. Leutz is primary author of three books on the practical development of coordinated community health care systems for elders.

Dr. Leutz can be contacted at the Schneider Institute for Health Policy, The Heller School, Mailstop 035, Waltham, MA 02454 (E-mail: leutz@brandeis.edu).

Merwyn Greenlick is Professor Emeritus and past chair of the Department of Public Health and Preventive Medicine, School of Medicine, Oregon Health & Sciences University. He also directs the Oregon Health Policy Institute. Until July 1995, he was Director of the Kaiser Permanente Center for Health Research (CHR) and Vice President for Research, Kaiser Foundation Hospitals. He was instrumental in starting the CHR in 1964 and was its director for more than 30 years. Dr. Greenlick's research has been in the areas of large-scale demonstration projects relating to the organization and financing of medical care and behavioral interventions in disease prevention. Dr. Greenlick is a Distinguished Fellow of the Association for Health Services Research (now the Academy for Health Services Research and Health Policy) and, in 1994, received the Association's President's Award for his lifetime contributions to the field.

Dr. Greenlick can be contacted at 712 NW Spring Ave., Portland, OR 97229.

Lucy Nonnenkamp is Project Director for the Kaiser Permanente Northwest's (KPNW) Social HMO, co-chairs KPNW's Senior and Disabled Care committee, and participates in the KPNW's Medicare visioning, strategic planning, oversight, and operations functions. She coordinated the 1996 Kaiser Permanente Interregional Geriatric Institute and is currently on the Kaiser Permanente Aging Network Advisory committee. Ms. Nonnenkamp was Project Administrator prior to becoming Project Director for the KPNW's Social HMO, locally marketed as Senior Advantage II.

Ms. Nonnenkamp can be contacted at Kaiser Center for Health Research, 2701 NW Vaughn St., Suite 160, Portland, OR 97210.

Dr. Richard della Penna is a geriatrician and is in his 25th year with Kaiser Permanente. He is the National Clinical Lead for Kaiser's Care Management Institute's Elder Care Initiative, and the national Director of the Kaiser Permanente Aging Network. His research and focus have been on the needs of older adults with dementia, depression, frailty, and those with advanced illness. He has published widely on dementia care, interdisciplinary team training, end of life care, integrating acute and long-term care, and Medicare managed care.

Dr. della Penna can be contacted at Kaiser Permanente Aging Network, 10992 San Diego Mission Road, San Diego, CA 92108.

REFERENCES

Brody, K. et al. (1997). Evaluation of a self-report screening instrument to predict frailty outcomes in aging populations. *The Gerontologist, 37*(2), 182-191.

Greenlick, M. R. et al. (1988). The S/HMO Demonstration: Policy implications for long-term care in HMOs. *Pride Institute Journal, 7*(3), 15-24.

Kramer, A. M. et al. (1992). Geriatric care approaches in health maintenance organizations. *J. of the Amer Ger Assoc, 40*, 1055-1067.

Kutza, E. (1997). Implications of an aging society for the organization and evaluation of public health services. *Public Health and Aging.* T. Hickey, M. Speers, and T. Prohaska (Eds.). Baltimore: The Johns Hopkins University Press, 293-308.

Leutz, W. (1999). Five laws for integrating medical and social care: Lessons from the US and UK. *The Milbank Memorial Fund Quarterly, 77*(1), 77-110.

Leutz, W. et al. (1994). Integrating acute and long-term care. *Health Affairs* (Fall).

Leutz, W. et al. (2002). *Kaiser Permanente's Manifesto 2005 Demonstration: The Promises and Limits of Devolutions.* Portland, OR: Kaiser Permanente Center for Health Research.

Marshall, B. et al. (1999). Case management of the elderly in a HMO: The implications for program administration under managed care. *Journal of Healthcare Management, 44*(6), 477-491.

Splaine, M. et al. (1998). Implementing a strategy for improving care: Lessons from studying those age 80 and older in a health system. *Journal of Ambulatory Care Management, 21*(3), 56-59.

Wiener, J., & Skaggs, J. (1995). *Current Approaches to Integrating Acute and LTC Financing and Services.* Washington, DC: AARP Public Policy Institute.

Age Concerns:
Innovation Through Care Management

David Stoesz, PhD

Virginia Commonwealth University

SUMMARY. Age Concerns is a proprietary care management firm serving the elderly. Established in 1982, the firm has prospered by employing an integrated model of care whereby the caregivers are employees of Age Concerns. In addition, the firm's ability to keep the elderly at home, out of institutional care, has resonated with consumers. Various features of Age Concerns–organizational format, characteristics of consumers, and economic considerations–are described. In 2001, Age Concerns was acquired by the Senior Care Action Network, a social health maintenance organization. In an increasingly commercial environment in which the elderly are a burgeoning market, Age Concerns may be a prototype of future elder-care service delivery. *[Article copies available for a fee from The Haworth Document Delivery Service: 1-800-HAWORTH. E-mail address: <getinfo@haworthpressinc.com> Website: <http://www.HaworthPress.com> © 2002 by The Haworth Press, Inc. All rights reserved.]*

KEYWORDS. Home care, proprietary (for-profit) human services, innovations in elder care

INTRODUCTION

In 1982, B. J. Curry Spitler, a social policy professor, responded to a young psychiatrist's query about an elderly, alcoholic couple "whose lives were out of control." Employing a social work approach, she as-

[Haworth co-indexing entry note]: "Age Concerns: Innovation Through Care Management." Stoesz, David. Co-published simultaneously in *Journal of Aging & Social Policy* (The Haworth Press, Inc.) Vol. 14, No. 3/4, 2002, pp. 245-260; and: *Devolution and Aging Policy* (ed: Francis G. Caro, and Robert Morris) The Haworth Press, Inc., 2002, pp. 245-260. Single or multiple copies of this article are available for a fee from The Haworth Document Delivery Service [1-800-HAWORTH, 9:00 a.m. - 5:00 p.m. (EST). E-mail address: getinfo@haworthpressinc.com].

10.1300/J031v14n03_14

sessed their problems, negotiated a care plan with their adult children, and hired attendants to care for them. Not long thereafter, Spitler had received a third, then a fourth referral. By 1985, the number of cases reached 18, necessitating the acquisition of support staff as well as more suitable office space. Spitler soon left her university post in order to devote time to her new firm, Age Concerns, Inc. Fifteen years later, the San Diego care management firm served 140 clients and employed 200 staff, boasting an annual budget of $5 million (Spitler, *Origins*).

The success of Age Concerns reflects the convergence of several vectors in human services: an increase of affluent elders who can afford intensive care, a recognition of the detrimental affects of nursing home care, a demand for alternatives to traditional institutional care, and the proliferation of proprietary firms providing care for the aged. As the nation anticipates a spike in the number of older Americans during the coming decades, innovations such as Age Concerns warrant examination.

THE CONTEXT

Prior to the Social Security Act, care of the elderly was a responsibility of family and community. The 1935 Social Security Act provided the infrastructure for federal social programs that have evolved to serve the elderly. Meager cash welfare provided by Old Age Assistance was soon eclipsed by social insurance benefits of Social Security. Despite the enormous popularity of Social Security, it failed to address health care, an omission corrected in part with the passage of Medicare and Medicaid. Yet, the 1965 health care amendments to the Social Security Act would prove problematic: Medicare, noted the founder of Age Concerns, does not cover long-term care, yet it is long-term custodial and supportive care that most older people need in order to maintain themselves in their homes and to preserve their autonomy and sense of independence. Those 85 and older make up the fastest growing segment of our aging population. This group is three times as likely to suffer from chronic illness and have significant deficits in their activities of daily living as the groups from 65 to 85. When chronic illness is not attended to with supportive care, it can become catastrophic illness, which requires more intensive care, meaning institutionalization and dramatically increased costs (Spitler, *Origins*, p. 3).

Since Medicare focused on acute care and Medicaid covered long-term care, those elders who might have been maintained independently at home were often sent to nursing homes instead, a fate which necessitated destitution since Medicaid was means-tested. Medicare and Medicaid thus launched the American health care industry, one organized around institutional care. Not surprisingly, its first institutional manifestation was the for-profit nursing home, a model that soon dominated elder care. "Given the rapid growth of an extensive nursing home system with large capital investments and ideological and practice links to medicine," reflected Morris, Caro, and Hansan, "efforts concentrated initially on controls in nursing homes rather than alternative care modalities" (1998, p. 13). Initial enthusiasm for home care as a substitute for nursing homes foundered on government reports questioning cost savings. Regardless, the promise of Medicare reimbursement propelled a burgeoning home care industry, until a 1997 federal audit revealed that as much as 40% of the charges were unjustified (Pear, 1997; Havemann, 1997). Medicare payments for home health peaked in 1996 at $18.1 billion, subsequently plummeting to $9.3 billion in 1999 (U.S. House Ways and Means Committee, 2000, p. 134).

The disconnection between Medicare and Medicaid required millions of older Americans to "spend-down" their assets to qualify for Medicaid. In the absence of alternatives to institutionalization, pauperization became the means to meet the soaring costs of nursing home care. Elders wanting to avoid nursing homes by remaining at home had little choice but to rely on a largely unregulated home care industry. Among the few credible innovations during the 1980s and 1990s was the deployment of a handful of Social Health Maintenance Organizations that integrated medical and social approaches to elder care.

Demographics drive social policy, and nowhere is this more evident than in care of the aged. With the new millennium, 35 million Americans were over 65 years of age, a number expected to double by 2030. While some older Americans remain poor, the median net worth of households headed by elders increased 70% between 1984 and 1999; the median net worth of white households was $181,000 in 1999. With increased longevity have come chronic health problems: 25% of the elderly suffer from some form of disability; of those 85 and older, 23% report severe depression and 36% evidence severe memory loss (*Older Americans 2000*); 75% have three or more deficits in daily living activities. Over 30% of people 65 and older live alone (Spitler, *Origins*, p. 4). Significantly, the number of older Americans in nursing homes has declined as has the number receiving care in the community. For those receiving home care, most of the care–64% in 1994–was exclusively informal and/or unpaid.

Logically, the demand for home health care increases with age: In 1998, the number of home health visits per 1,000 Medicare enrollees aged 65 to 74 was 2,350; for those 75 to 84, it was 6,262; for those 85 and older, it skyrocketed to 12,709. Although most home health care has been informal, reliance on professional assistance has increased as disability increases. Between 1982 and 1994, the percent of Medicare beneficiaries with five Activity in Daily Living (ADL) deficits and who receive a mix of informal and formal care increased from 33.2% to 55.3%. By comparison, the number receiving only formal care increased from only 1.5% to 3.3%. In 1994, 4.7 million Medicare beneficiaries received home health care for at least one ADL (Spitler, *Origins*, p. 4).

Policy and demographics have catalyzed a "gray market" in services to older Americans (Stoesz, 1990). Initially evident in nursing homes followed by home health agencies, the gray market has undergone considerable elaboration. Assisted living facilities have evolved to fill the niche between nursing homes and retirement centers, operated by corporations such as Alterra Healthcare Corporation (Meier, 2000). Assisted living provides residential care for elders who need help with daily living for fees ranging from $2,500 to $6,000 per month, most of which is paid out-of-pocket (Steinhauer, 2001). The services offered through assisted living are not well defined and vary considerably. While most residential fees cover maid service, special diets, and personal laundry, only half provide transportation, assistance with daily living, and medication administration; only one-third assure nursing services and incontinence care. As a result, supplemental fees are often levied, and these can be a burden, particularly since more than 90% are paid by self or family. Often, irregular billing for supplemental services has led to consumer complaints. When assisted living arrangements fail, most residents are placed in nursing homes (Goldstein, 2001a, 2001b).

CARE MANAGEMENT

The demand for high-quality care for older Americans has generated the specialization of "care management." That coordination of care would be necessary for elders who are experiencing multiple difficulties negotiating their environment is incontrovertible; yet, how that coordination occurs has important nuances. On behalf of the Health Resources and Services Administration of the Department of Health and Human Services, an interdisciplinary team defined care coordination as "case management."

Case management is a service that coordinates and links care across health and social service organizations, systems, and networks, within institutions and the community to locate and arrange necessary resources, equipment, and supplies from formal and informal sources including professionals, paraprofessionals, volunteers, family, and friends (Netting, 1995). Accordingly, the prudent case manager conducts a systematic assessment, develops, implements, and monitors a care plan, and discharges the client when appropriate.

The rapid expansion, then attenuation, of services by case management corporations have left the term with a negative connotation, however. As Spitler observed, case management has come to be understood as gatekeepers who ration services to consumers, effectively circumscribing the care that they need. Rather than attenuate care for the elderly, Spitler contended that providers should optimize services through "care management." She was clear about the contrast between "case management" and "care management": "Any successful policy must empower older people to choose among options and help them live out their lives with dignity" (Spitler, 1996, p. 170).

As emphasis on consumer choice shaped elder care, a network of managed care providers has evolved. Begun in 1989, the National Association of Professional Geriatric Care Managers (NAPGCM) has grown from 108 to 1,520 member organizations in 2001 (Rosenberg, 2001). The NAPGCM identifies seven activities that constitute care management:

- Biopsychosocial assessment
- Exploration of options and the development of a care plan
- Staffing
- Monitoring client progress and supportive supervision of attendants
- Activities management and service coordination
- Advocacy
- Record-keeping and case review (Spitler, 1996, p. 172).

Within care management, two models evolved, the brokerage model and the integrated model. "In the brokerage model, caregivers are not employed by the geriatric care management organization (GCM). The GCM assesses the client's level of functioning and living situation, explores options, develops a care plan, and either refers the client or arranges for services." By contrast, in the integrated model, caregivers are employed by the geriatric care management organization. The GCM assesses the client and the situation, explores options, and develops a plan of care. If caregiver, transportation, shopping, home repair, and other miscellaneous services are required, these resources are furnished by or through the GCM's organization. The GCM employs and monitors the caregivers providing services (Spitler & Hansen, 2001, p. 44).

Age Concerns[1]

As a provider of care management, Age Concerns grew as Spitler diligently cultivated client referrals, instituted sound business practices, acquired committed staff, and exploited linkages with community agencies. Some ventures proved challenging: When the local Housing Authority needed to relocate 40 seniors temporarily for apartment repairs, Age Concerns won a contract for which there had been little interest, bolstered staffing, and facilitated the transition. Others must have seemed Quixotic: When the California Thoroughbred Horsemen's Association asked for help with 34 jockeys, stable hands, and exercise boys who had not been particularly gracious about the prospects of retirement, Age Concerns eased the transition:

> They were a hard drinking rough living bunch of fellows. The Association had tried to contract with Adult Protective Services, but after a year APS had pronounced them noncompliant, uncooperative, and incorrigible and wanted no part of them. Age Concerns took them on and discovered that they were eligible for Medicaid, SSI, and other benefits. The Association had been paying for all other expenses. After Age Concerns got their benefits straightened out, the company were the "fair-haired children" for many years. Age Concerns provided full care management, saw that they had adequate housing, took them to the doctor, etc. When they died, Age Concerns arranged for their funerals and settled their small estates. (Spitler, 2001, p. 2)

Throughout, Spitler held to her beliefs that "relationships and autonomy are two of the most prized aspects of adult life," an orientation that doubtless resonated with the scruffy horsemen. "Our humanness is shaped by the relationships and social exchanges we negotiate daily. As autonomous adults we have the right to make our own decisions about what work we do, where to live, how to use our leisure, what religion to adopt, and which relationships to maintain. Successful aging can be considered the constructive use of autonomy throughout the life span" (Spitler, 2000, p. 2).

Services. Age Concerns provides three levels of care that are coordinated by care managers: homemaker services, personal care, and total care. Among care managers and caregivers, staff activities are roughly divided as follows: 12.5% for homemaker services, 50% for personal care, 25% for total care, and 12.5% for care management only. Client needs with respect to ADLs are extensive (Table 1).

ADL data fail to capture the affection on the part of caregivers for their clients, particularly those for whom care had been provided for years; nor do they reflect the appreciation of clients for services received. Three anecdotes are illustrative:

- A couple was having difficulty managing their affairs due to the wife's colon cancer and the husband's early stage of Alzheimer's disease. Their son and daughter-in-law had demanding professional careers and were raising two teenage sons. An Age Concerns care manager acted as an extension of the family to oversee every aspect of care for the parents: accompanying them on medical appointments, addressing the wife's alcoholism, arranging for the wife's funeral and memorial, assisting the husband attend to his vegetable garden, negotiating home repairs, and attending to his personal needs. After the husband's death, the son began his eulogy by thanking Age Concerns and each of the caregivers who had cared for his parents for six years: "It was Age Concerns' dedicated service that allowed us to fulfill our commitments to my parents–to insure that they received the absolute best care in their beloved home in Coronado–and yet still permit my wife and me to carry on a semblance of a normal life" (Spitler, *Origins*, pp. 9-10).
- A Latina caregiver of a university professor of Mexican art suffering from Alzheimer's disease cajoled the professor out of his

TABLE 1. Client ADL Needs

ADL	Percent Needing Assistance		
	Independent	Partial Assistance	Total Assistance
Bathing	47.4	27.9	16.2
Dressing	49.4	23.4	20.1
Grooming	44.2	16.2	15.6
Eating	74.7	14.9	3.2
Oral hygiene	62.3	14.3	12.3
Toileting	61.0	16.2	13.6

wheelchair by offering to dance with him. "You know, he was quite a lady's man, at one time," she said, leading her client through an attenuated two-step. "This is about the only way I can get him up on his feet. He doesn't respond to much anymore, but sometimes he'll talk back when I speak to him in Spanish."

- Another caregiver was assigned to a retired biology teacher who had been an avid hiker but now suffers from advanced Alzheimer's. "When I came here eight years ago, I didn't know what to do because she didn't want to have me around," admitted the caregiver. "But she would go out for these long walks and get lost, and it was dangerous for her. So, I just told her, 'Pretend that I'm your puppy following you around' [pantomiming panting with hands flopped at her chest], and she accepted that. Wheew! For the next years, did I get a work out–we hiked all over! I can't tell you how much she taught me."[2]

The duration of services varied considerably, ranging from one month to 14 years. On average, the length of service provision was four years.

Clientele. The clients of Age Concerns mirror the attributes of older Americans: three-fourths are women, and half are widowed. Most are advanced in their years (Table 2).

Two-thirds of clients own homes or condos, while 7% live in apartments, 9.5% in assisted living facilities, 7.9% in a skilled nursing facilities, and 5.5% in board and care homes. Many have been determined to be unable to manage their affairs: 17.6% have a conservator, and the bills of 24.2% are paid by a trust officer. Because Age Concerns does not accept payment from Medicare or Medicaid, clients must be reasonably affluent to afford care; during the first two weeks of 2001, the average bill was $1,461.72, while the median bill was $634.85. On average, the monthly revenue derived per client is $5,000, significantly less than typical nursing home costs which are 50% higher.[3] Approximately 47% of clients are billed for hourly services, 24% for live-in services, and 8% for 10- to 12-hour shifts.

Clients of Age Concerns present various problems that complicate their care. For example, 24.7% are incontinent. Debilitating medical conditions are prevalent: 31.2% evidence heart disease, 16.2% arthritis, 12.3% stroke, 7.8% cancer, 7.1% fractures, and 3.9% Parkinson's disease. In addition, 56.9% suffer from cognitive impairment, aside from various mental health conditions (see Table 3).

Staff. Age Concerns subscribes to an "integrated model" of care management, employing the coordinators as well as the caregivers. Spitler

TABLE 2. Age of Clients

Age	Number	%
Under 60	6	3.8
60-64	1	0.6
65-69	5	3.2
70-74	11	7.1
75-79	19	12.3
80-84	30	19.5
85-89	35	22.7
90-94	38	24.7
95-99	5	3.2
Over 100	4	2.6

has been adamant about clients retaining their freedom and therein control over their environment: "The mission of Age Concerns is to enhance the lives of our clients to the maximum extent possible by fostering the older person's health, self-esteem and right to self-determination" (Age Concerns, 2000). A Director of Clinical Services oversees one Clinical Supervisor, eight professional Care Managers, and one Intake Coordinator. Care Managers coordinate the service of 200 full- and part-time Care-Givers, who served 175 clients in December 2001 (Spitler, 2000, p. 2). Age Concerns prides itself on having experienced, professional Care Managers, staff possessing Masters of Social Work or Registered Nurse credentials. The salary of Care Managers ranges from $40,000 to $50,000 annually. Care Managers are loyal employees; turnover in 1999 was 20%, considerably lower than that of agencies in the region, where 40% to 60% turnovers were common.

Care-Givers are less-credentialed, but receive eight hours of orientation and training before being dispatched to serve clients. Training includes orientation to company policies, procedures, and benefits; Universal Safety Standards in compliance with OSHA; Dementia Care Training; and Companion Care Training. Care-Givers are perceived as integral to the Age Concerns "family" and are rewarded accordingly: hourly wages average $10.00; Care-Givers are paid about $100 for each shift of extended or live-in care. Care-Givers are provided with health benefits and are offered a 401(k) benefit, although their contributions are not matched. Among full-time Care-Givers, turnover was 34.8% in 1999 and 30.3% in 2000; for part-time Care-Givers, turnover was 49.1% and

TABLE 3. Client Mental Disorders

Disorder	Prevalence in %
Dementia	54.3
Confusion	42.5
Memory loss	49.7
Impaired judgment	40.5
Anxiety	28.1
Paranoia	13.8
Depression	25.5
Alcohol abuse	9.2

32.2%, respectively. The turnover of Age Concerns Care-Givers compares favorably to the 50% to 70% turnover typical of providers in the region that employ staff. Spitler attributes Age Concerns' relatively low Care-Giver turnover to above market average wages and a benefits package that includes health and dental care and a retirement plan that is available after a year of service.

The recruitment and retention of Care-Givers is the responsibility of a Human Resource Manager who supervises two full-time coordinators. Although the region has had a tight labor market, "Age Concerns has been able to retain highly qualified, dedicated Care-Givers." Because Care-Givers are the most conspicuous representative of Age Concerns, the company frequently reminds them of their importance. "They are the eyes and ears, heart and hands of the organization in providing care for the elderly," noted Spitler. "The Care-Givers are counseled that every employee projects the image of Age Concerns, and it is the responsibility of each person to project an image congruent with our mission" (Spitler, 2000, p. 7). Spitler observes that the careful matching of Care-Givers to clients is the key to Care-Giver retention *and* client satisfaction.

Structure. The structure of any organization reflects authority in decision-making as well as a balance in task responsibilities. As depicted by its organizational chart (Figure 1), Age Concerns employs a Board of Directors, chaired by the company's founder, who advises the Chief Executive Officer, the founder's daughter, who oversees six division heads: Clinical Services, Sales, Human Resources, Controller, Marketing, and the Office Manager. These divisions have evolved over time, though Clinical Services, Human Resources, and Controller divisions have been the core of the company.

The balance of task responsibilities helps explain the company's success. The Clinical Director supervises eight Care Managers who coordinate the care for no more than 20 clients. For the first three quarters of 2000, Age Concerns cared for 143 clients, accepting eight new clients each month. During this period the number of administrative and professional staff (management and Care Managers) numbered 25, while the number of Care-Givers numbered 162. Since most activity consists of direct client care, most of Age Concerns' budget is dedicated accordingly: for 2000, 89.2% was allocated for Care-Givers and 10.8% for Care Management.

Finances. An increasingly competitive human services environment highlights the role of finance in service delivery. Since most activity consists of direct client care, most of Age Concerns' budget is dedicated accordingly: for 2000, 72% of the firm's $5.4 million in revenues were allocated for Care-Giver and Care Management compensation and benefits. Having become established as a primary provider of care management in an expanding market, Age Concerns anticipates significant growth in sales over the next three years. Over that period, the firm expects to increase its annual revenues by about 80%. Because of this growth in revenue and achieving certain economies of scale, Age Concerns expects to more than double its annual gross profits during this same period.

Client Satisfaction. When clients have a choice in service provision, companies cannot afford to be negligent with respect to consumer perceptions of the care they receive. To determine consumer satisfaction, Age Concerns crafted a satisfaction questionnaire, modeled after existing instruments (Smith, 2000). The questionnaire was mailed to "clients" or, because a sizable subset suffered from cognitive impairments and conservators had been designated to manage their affairs, "collaterals." Of the 67 surveys sent to clients, 31 were returned; of 136 questionnaires mailed to collaterals, 55 responded.

Regardless of the respondent being a client or collateral, responses were uniformly positive, often in the 80 and 90 percentiles. For example, 93% of clients and 96% of collaterals were "very or mostly satisfied" with services received. When asked "to what extent has our program met your needs?" 100% of clients and 98% of collaterals responded affirmatively. Ninety-seven percent of clients and 96% of collaterals said they would recommend the program to a friend in need of similar help. There was a subtle pattern in responses: Those nearest to the client

FIGURE 1. Age Concerns Organizational Chart (1/8/01)

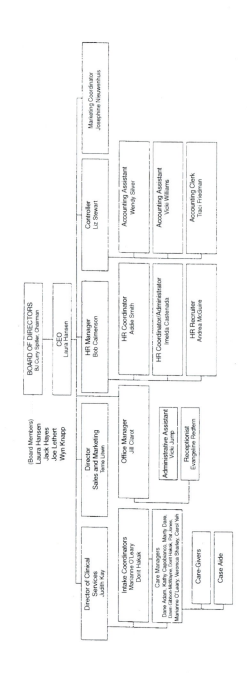

256

received higher marks; Care-Givers ranked a bit higher than Care Managers, and Care Managers rated higher than office staff, but even then, all responses were positive, above 50%. When queried about their decision in selecting Age Concerns as a provider, 93% of clients and 93% of collaterals stated they were confident they had made the right decision. Similarly, when asked if consideration was being given to changing to a different service provider, 96% of clients and 98% of collaterals responded negatively.

THE FUTURE OF AGE CONCERNS

In 2000, Age Concerns began negotiations with the Senior Care Action Network (SCAN), a southern California social health maintenance organization. Since its authorization in 1984, SCAN had become a major service provider to elders, by 2000 subscribing 47,626 members, building a staff of 580, and accruing a budget of $342 million. While traditional HMOs aggressively pursued Medicare beneficiaries, then threatened to dump them when reimbursement fell short of corporate expectations, SCAN's founder and director Sam Ervin maintained an even course, insisting that SCAN honor its "commitment to help seniors receive quality benefits at a reasonable cost" (SCAN, p. 1). In 2001, SCAN acquired Age Concerns as a vehicle to extend provision of care management.

Age Concerns became a regional leader in elder care because founder B. J. Spitler and CEO Laura Hansen had assiduously cultivated its "niche" (Spitler & Hansen, 2001, p. 43). They believed that collaborating with SCAN would disseminate the model they had perfected. As a nonprofit organization, SCAN wanted to acquire a commercial unit that could generate capital while providing high quality service. Despite their for-profit/nonprofit differences, the organizations complement each other in an important way. As opposed to the dominant medical model that had defined care for the aged since the passage of Medicare and Medicaid, Age Concerns and SCAN opted for an integrated model that employs care managers to match caregivers with clients who need help with a range of needs, from household modification to personal assistance (Morris, Caro, & Hansan, 1998).

While the SCAN/Age Concerns collaboration may bode well for the elderly in southern California, a larger policy question looms: how to integrate a social model of care management with a medical model that has defined elder care for three decades? The inherent limits of Medicare and Medicaid are well known: the former, an insurance program for the elderly who experience acute illness; the latter, public assistance for the poor who need long-term care. Compounding the social insurance versus public assistance problem has been a fundamental structural difference: Medicare is a universal program operated uniformly across the nation, while Medicaid evidences the vicissitudes associated with a collaboration between state and federal governments. Adding to these structural problems an impending inundation of health care needs from aging baby boomers quite literally explodes the integrity of current health policy.

Fading enthusiasm for a unified solution to the nation's health care needs, such as the single-payer model, has focused attention away from entities that are national and public and toward those that are local and private. Here, a dynamic and expanding health care industry has emerged, the power of which was evident when the Health Security Act was dispensed with in 1993. The reconciliation of these altogether different entities has proven awkward. In 1999 Medicare+Choice was introduced, and 260 HMOs contracted to subscribe Medicare beneficiaries (U.S. House Ways and Means Committee, 2000, pp. 1182-1218); however, problems soon surfaced with the threatened termination of thousands of elders who had switched from fee-for-service to managed care. In 2001, the Bush administration proposed to further fragment health financing with the introduction of Medical Savings Accounts.

It is within the burgeoning service sector of a post-industrial society that Age Concerns is best appreciated. An industrial order that gave rise to the public bureaucracies of the welfare state has been eclipsed by a new era in which the private sector has become the fount of innovation in human service provision. This shift is of tectonic magnitude since it occurs as an enormous cohort of baby boomers is approaching retirement and the eventual need for long-term care. Clearly, traditional solutions to this problem do not suffice. "A social insurance model that would provide universal or near universal coverage for some aspect of long-term care is highly unlikely in the current political climate," observed Morris, Caro, and Hansan (1998, p. 163). At the same time, proposals by the Bush administration to restructure Medicare and privatize Social Security suggest that modification of these essential programs may be forthcoming. If social insurance for the elderly is reformed, prospects brighten for private sector innovations that have served a larger social purpose. In that event, the virtues of a hybrid medical/social model of care management may well elevate Age Concerns as an exemplar in elder care.

NOTES

1. The description of Age Concerns is derived from company records, interviews with administrators, care managers, and clients in January 2001.
2. A similarly touching account of the relationship between elder and caregiver appears in Abel and Nelson (2001).
3. Approximation based on average daily Medicare payments to skilled nursing facilities of $250 during the late 1990s (U.S. House Ways and Means Committee, 2000, p. 130).

AUTHOR NOTES

David Stoesz is Professor of Social Policy at the Northern Virginia Social Work Program of Virginia Commonwealth University in Arlington, Virginia. He is (co)author of books on social policy, welfare reform, child protection, and international development. Currently, Dr. Stoesz is writing a book on theory and social policy.

Dr. Stoesz can be contacted at Virginia Commonwealth University, School of Social Work, 3330 Washington Blvd., Arlington, VA 22201 (E-mail: dstoesz@mail1.vcu.edu).

REFERENCES

Abel, M., & Nelson, M. (2001). Intimate care for hire. *The American Prospect*, May 21.

Age Concerns (2000). Company description. San Diego, CA.

Goldstein, A. (2001a, February 19). Assisted living: helping hand may not be enough. *Washington Post*.

Goldstein, A. (2001b, February 20). Assisted living: paying the price. *Washington Post*.

Havemann, J. (1997, July 29). Fraud rife in elder home care. *Washington Post*.

Meier, B. (2000, November 25). States see problems with care at chain of centers for aged. *New York Times*.

Morris, R., Caro, F., & Hansan, J. (1998). *Personal Assistance: The Future of Home Care*. Baltimore: Johns Hopkins University Press.

Netting, F. (1995). Case management, in S. Klein (Ed.), *The National Forum on Geriatric Education and Training*. Washington, DC: U.S. Department of Health and Human Services.

Older Americans 2000: Key Indicators of Well-Being, http://www.agingstats.gov/chartbook2000/aboutthisreport/html.

Pear, R. (1997, July 27). Investigators say a Medicare option is rife with fraud. *New York Times*.

Rosenberg, C. (2001). Personal correspondence March 12. National Association of Geriatric Care Management, Services and Resources for Seniors, Inc., 930 Mt. Kemble Ave., Morristown, NJ.

SCAN (no date). Committed to . . . passion, integrity, respect, and responsibility. Long Beach, CA.

Smith, M. (2000). Satisfaction, in R. Kane and R. Kane (Eds.), *Assessing Older Persons*. New York: Oxford University Press.

Spitler, B. J. (2001). *My Memoirs*. San Diego: author.

Spitler, B. J. (2000). Age concerns. SCAN. Long Beach, CA, July 27.

Spitler, B. J. (1996). A social work perspective of care management, in S. Blancett and D. Flarey (Eds.), *Case Studies in Nursing Care Management*. Gaithersburg, MD: Aspen Publishers.

Spitler, B. J. (no date). *Origins of Age Concerns*. San Diego: author.

Spitler, B. J., & Hansen, L. (2001). After the start-up: issues for mature care management organizations, in C. Cress, (Ed.), *Handbook of Geriatric Care Management*. Gaithersburg, MD.

Steinhauer, J. (2001, February 12). As assisted living centers grow, calls for standards and oversight. *New York Times*.

Stoesz, D. (1990). The gray market. *Journal of Gerontological Social Work*, January.

U.S. House Ways and Means Committee (2000). *Overview of Entitlement Programs*. Washington, DC.

Index